The 5th International Congress of CiiEM — Reducing inequalities in Health and Society

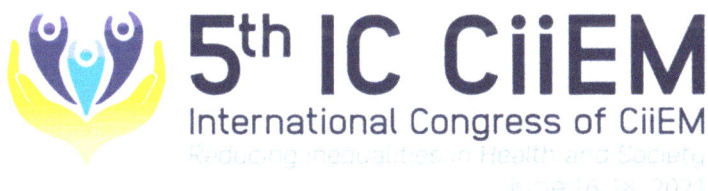

The 5th International Congress of CiiEM—Reducing inequalities in Health and Society

Editors

Helena Barroso
Cidália Castro

MDPI • Basel • Beijing • Wuhan • Barcelona • Belgrade

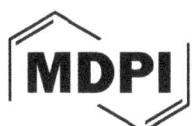

Editors
Helena Barroso
Instituto Universitário Egas Moniz
Portugal

Cidália Castro
Instituto Universitário Egas Moniz
Portugal

Editorial Office
MDPI
St. Alban-Anlage 66
4052 Basel, Switzerland

This is a reprint of articles from the Conference Proceedings published online in the open access journal *Medical Sciences* (ISSN 2076-3271) from 2021 (available at: https://www.mdpi.com/2673-9992/5/1).

For citation purposes, cite each article independently as indicated on the article page online and as indicated below:

LastName, A.A.; LastName, B.B.; LastName, C.C. Article Title. *Journal Name* **Year**, *Article Number*, Page Range.

ISBN 978-3-0365-2237-1 (Pbk)
ISBN 978-3-0365-2238-8 (PDF)

Cover image courtesy of Egas Moniz, CRL

© 2021 by the authors. Articles in this book are Open Access and distributed under the Creative Commons Attribution (CC BY) license, which allows users to download, copy and build upon published articles, as long as the author and publisher are properly credited, which ensures maximum dissemination and a wider impact of our publications.

The book as a whole is distributed by MDPI under the terms and conditions of the Creative Commons license CC BY-NC-ND.

Contents

About the Editors xi

Preface to "The 5th International Congress of CiiEM—Reducing inequalities in Health and Society" xiii

Beatriz Setoca and Ana I. Fernandes
Dispensing of Food Supplements in the Treatment and Prevention of Urinary Tract Infections
Reprinted from: *Medical Sciences Forum* **2021**, *5*, 1, doi:10.3390/msf2021005001 1

Nuno F. da Costa, João F. Pinto and Ana I. Fernandes
Cohesiveness of Powdered Co-Amorphous Olanzapine and Impact on Tablet Production
Reprinted from: *Medical Sciences Forum* **2021**, *5*, 2, doi:10.3390/msf2021005002 5

Joana Macedo, Valérie Vanhoorne, Chris Vervaet and João F. Pinto
Can Fused Deposition Modelling Enable the Manufacture of Uniform and Precise Dose Tablets?
Reprinted from: *Medical Sciences Forum* **2021**, *5*, 3, doi:10.3390/msf2021005003 9

Maria D. Auxtero, Mário Abade, Susana Chalante, Bianca Silva and Ana I. Fernandes
Nutraceuticals for Smart Aging and Potential Drug Interactions
Reprinted from: *Medical Sciences Forum* **2021**, *5*, 4, doi:10.3390/msf2021005004 11

Josefa Domingos, Tamine Capato and Catarina Godinho
The Profile of People with Parkinson's Disease Included in Community Boxing Exercise Programs
Reprinted from: *Medical Sciences Forum* **2021**, *5*, 5, doi:10.3390/msf2021005005 13

João Gato Marques, Cecília Rozan, Luís Proença, André Peixoto and Cristina Manso
Assessment of Hyposalivation, Xerostomia, and Oral Health-Related Quality of Life in Polymedicated Patients
Reprinted from: *Medical Sciences Forum* **2021**, *5*, 6, doi:10.3390/msf2021005006 17

Sofia Santos, Paulo Mascarenhas, Susana Bandarra, Ana Clara Ribeiro, Paulo Maurício and Isabel Barahona
Evaluation of the Cytotoxic Potential of Adhesives, with Two on the Market: Scotchbond Universal and Optibond Solo Plus, and an Adhesive in the Experimental Phase: T1
Reprinted from: *Medical Sciences Forum* **2021**, *5*, 7, doi:10.3390/msf2021005007 21

Inês Caetano Santos, Fabrícia Martins, Kateryna Rudysh, Luís Proença, Ana Cristina Manso, Mário Polido, José João Mendes and Helena Canhão
Xerostomia and Medication in an Elderly Portuguese Population
Reprinted from: *Medical Sciences Forum* **2021**, *5*, 8, doi:10.3390/msf2021005008 25

Catarina Izidoro, João Botelho, Vanessa Machado, Luis Proença, Ricardo Alves and José João Mendes
Halitosis Self-Perception and Awareness among Periodontal Patients—An Exploratory Study
Reprinted from: *Medical Sciences Forum* **2021**, *5*, 9, doi:10.3390/msf2021005009 27

Catarina Egreja and Noémia Lopes
Students, Medicines and Performance Consumption: The Online as a Source of Information and Sharing
Reprinted from: *Medical Sciences Forum* **2021**, *5*, 10, doi:10.3390/msf2021005010 29

Inês Teodoro, Hugo Torres, Nuno Venâncio, Guilhermina Moutinho and Maria Deolinda Auxtero
Application of Cannabis Use Intention Questionnaire (CUIQ) to First Year University Students
Reprinted from: *Medical Sciences Forum* **2021**, *5*, 11, doi:10.3390/msf2021005011 33

Iris Almeida, Ana Rita Pires, Carolina Nobre, Joana Marques and Patrícia Oliveira
Intimate Partner Violence Risk Assessment in Victims Information and Assistance Office
Reprinted from: *Medical Sciences Forum* **2021**, *5*, 12, doi:10.3390/msf2021005012 37

Iris Almeida, Ana Ramalho, Joana Costa and Ricardo Ventura Baúto
The Forensic Psychology Role: Technical Advisor Office
Reprinted from: *Medical Sciences Forum* **2021**, *5*, 13, doi:10.3390/msf2021005013 39

Teresa Nascimento, João Inácio, Isabel Ferreira, Priscila Diaz, Paulo Freitas and Helena Barroso
Candida spp. Colonization among Intensive Care Unit Patients, Preliminary Results
Reprinted from: *Medical Sciences Forum* **2021**, *5*, 14, doi:10.3390/msf2021005014 41

Nuno Venâncio, Gabriela G. Pereira, João F. Pinto and Ana I. Fernandes
Influence of the Infill Geometry of 3D-Printed Tablets on Drug Dissolution
Reprinted from: *Medical Sciences Forum* **2021**, *5*, 15, doi:10.3390/msf2021005015 43

Diogo Sousa-Catita, Catarina Godinho and Jorge Fonseca
A Protocol for the Evaluation of Nutritional and Functional Status Evolution During a Multidisciplinary RehabilitationProgram for Patients after SARS-CoV-2 Pneumonia
Reprinted from: *Medical Sciences Forum* **2021**, *5*, 16, doi:10.3390/msf2021005016 47

Sara Figueiredo, João F. Pinto, Fátima G. Carvalho and Ana I. Fernandes
Tuning of Paroxetine 3D-Printable Formulations for Fused Deposition Modelling
Reprinted from: *Medical Sciences Forum* **2021**, *5*, 17, doi:10.3390/msf2021005017 51

Ricardo Ventura Baúto, Ana Filipa Carreiro, Margarida Pereira, Renata Guarda and Iris Almeida
Personality and Aggressive Behavior: The Relation between the Five-Factor and Aggression Models in a Domestic Violence Suspects Sample
Reprinted from: *Medical Sciences Forum* **2021**, *5*, 18, doi:10.3390/msf2021005018 53

Adriana M. L. Ferraz, Susana Bandarra, Paulo Mascarenhas, Isabel Barahona, Rui Martins and Ana Clara Ribeiro
Characterization of CYP2C19*17 Polymorphism in a Portuguese Population Sample Relevant for Proton Pump Inhibitor Therapy—A Pilot Study
Reprinted from: *Medical Sciences Forum* **2021**, *5*, 19, doi:10.3390/msf2021005019 55

Ana Raquel Barata, Gunel Kizi, Luis Proença, Valter Alves and Ana Sintra Delgado
Mouth Breathing and Atypical Swallowing in Adult Orthodontic Patients at Egas Moniz Dental Clinic: A Pilot Study
Reprinted from: *Medical Sciences Forum* **2021**, *5*, 20, doi:10.3390/msf2021005020 59

Violeta Alarcão, Pedro Candeias, Sónia Pintassilgo and Fernando Luís Machado
Exploring Inequalities in HPV Vaccine Uptake among Cape Verdean Immigrant and Portuguese Native Women
Reprinted from: *Medical Sciences Forum* **2021**, *5*, 21, doi:10.3390/msf2021005021 61

Paula Moleirinho-Alves, Pedro Cebola, André Almeida, Haúla Haider and João Paço
Treatment of Patients with Somatic Tinnitus Attributed to Temporomandibular Disorder: A Case Report
Reprinted from: *Medical Sciences Forum* **2021**, 5, 22, doi:10.3390/msf2021005022 65

Raquel Pacheco, Maria Alzira Cavacas, Paulo Mascarenhas, Pedro Oliveira and Carlos Zagalo
Incidence of OralMucositis in Patients Undergoing Head and Neck Cancer Treatment: Systematic Review andMeta-Analysis
Reprinted from: *Medical Sciences Forum* **2021**, 5, 23, doi:10.3390/msf2021005023 67

Juliana Pereira, Gunel Kizi, Ana Raquel Barata and Irene Ventura
Children's Oral Health on Pico Island, Azores (Portugal)
Reprinted from: *Medical Sciences Forum* **2021**, 5, 24, doi:10.3390/msf2021005024 69

Ana Sofia Alves, Gunel Kizi, Ana Raquel Barata, Paulo Mascarenhas and Irene Ventura
Oral Complications of Chemotherapy on Paediatric Patients with Cancer: A Systematic Review and Meta-Analysis
Reprinted from: *Medical Sciences Forum* **2021**, 5, 25, doi:10.3390/msf2021005025 71

Mariana Morgado, José João Mendes and Luís Proença
COVID-19 Risk Perception and Confidence among Clinical Dental Students: Impact on Patient Management
Reprinted from: *Medical Sciences Forum* **2021**, 5, 26, doi:10.3390/msf2021005026 73

Ana Sofia Pintado, Duarte Sousa-Tavares and Patrícia Cavaco-Silva
Awareness and Use of Heat-Not-Burn Tobacco among Students of Egas Moniz—Cooperative of Higher Education
Reprinted from: *Medical Sciences Forum* **2021**, 5, 27, doi:10.3390/msf2021005027 75

Miguel Grunho, Catarina Godinho, Marta Patita, Irina Mocanu, Ana Isabel Vieira, António Alves de Matos, Ricardo Carregosa, Frederico Marx, Morgane Tomé, Diogo Sousa-Catita, Luís Proença, Tiago Outeiro and Jorge Fonseca
Inflammatory Bowel Disease, Alpha-Synuclein Aggregates and Parkinson's Disease: The InflamaSPark Protocol
Reprinted from: *Medical Sciences Forum* **2021**, 5, 28, doi:10.3390/msf2021005028 77

Miguel Grunho, Catarina Godinho, Diogo Sousa-Catita, Filipa Vicente, Luís Proença, Ricardo Carregosa, Frederico Marx, Morgane Tomé, Josefa Domingos and Jorge Fonseca
Nutritional and Motor Functional Status in Parkinson's Disease: The NutriSPark Protocol
Reprinted from: *Medical Sciences Forum* **2021**, 5, 29, doi:10.3390/msf2021005029 79

Ana V. Antunes, Patrícia Oliveira, Jorge Cardoso and Telma C. Almeida
Adverse Childhood Experiences and Empathy: The Role of Interparental Conflict
Reprinted from: *Medical Sciences Forum* **2021**, 5, 30, doi:10.3390/msf2021005030 81

Miguel Grunho, Catarina Godinho, António Alves de Matos, Helena Barroso, Ricardo Carregosa, Frederico Marx, Morgane Tomé, Josefa Domingos, Diogo Sousa-Catita, João Botelho, Vanessa Machado, José João Mendes, Tiago Outeiro and Jorge Fonseca
Gut Status in Parkinson's Disease: The GutSPark Protocol
Reprinted from: *Medical Sciences Forum* **2021**, 5, 31, doi:10.3390/msf2021005031 83

Maria Santo, Maria D. Auxtero, Alexandra Figueiredo and Isabel Margarida Costa
Cow's Milk Protein Allergy: The Hidden Danger of Medicines' Excipients
Reprinted from: *Medical Sciences Forum* **2021**, 5, 32, doi:10.3390/msf2021005032 87

Sérgio Valério and Maria João Hilário
Patient Compliance with Oral Anticoagulant Therapy
Reprinted from: *Medical Sciences Forum* **2021**, *5*, 33, doi:10.3390/msf2021005033 89

Patrícia Cavaco-Silva, Maria Mole, Beatriz Meliço and Helena Barroso
S. aureus and MRSA Nasal Carriage in Dental Students: A Comprehensive Approach
Reprinted from: *Medical Sciences Forum* **2021**, *5*, 34, doi:10.3390/msf2021005034 91

Pedro Gameiro, Bernardo Saldanha, Francisco Santos, Jéssica Silva, João Norte, João Reis, Pedro Sottomayor, Rodolfo Vaz and Pedro Rodrigues
External Approach to Bilaterally Septated Maxillary Sinuses: A Case Report
Reprinted from: *Medical Sciences Forum* **2021**, *5*, 35, doi:10.3390/msf2021005035 93

Rodolfo Vaz, Pedro Gameiro, Pedro Sottomayor, Bernardo Saldanha and Pedro Rodrigues
Autologous Graft in the Anterior Maxilla—A Case Report
Reprinted from: *Medical Sciences Forum* **2021**, *5*, 36, doi:10.3390/msf2021005036 95

João Belo, André Almeida, Paula Moleirinho-Alves and Catarina Godinho
Temporomandibular Disorders and Bruxism Prevalence in a Portuguese Sample
Reprinted from: *Medical Sciences Forum* **2021**, *5*, 37, doi:10.3390/msf2021005037 97

Daniela Guerreiro, Ana Luísa Costa, Teresa Nascimento, Ana Clara Ribeiro, Luís Proença, José João Mendes and Helena Barroso
Massive Testing Is Important to Control a SARS-CoV-2 Outbreak
Reprinted from: *Medical Sciences Forum* **2021**, *5*, 38, doi:10.3390/msf2021005038 99

Susana Bandarra, Lurdes Monteiro and Laura Brum
Detection of the SARS-CoV-2 UK Variant in Portugal
Reprinted from: *Medical Sciences Forum* **2021**, *5*, 39, doi:10.3390/msf2021005039 101

Carolina Fernandes, Inês Allen, Leonor Sá Pinto, André Júdice, Filipa Vicente, Carlos Família, José João Mendes and Catarina Godinho
Oral Health among Athletes at the Egas Moniz Sports Dentistry Practice
Reprinted from: *Medical Sciences Forum* **2021**, *5*, 40, doi:10.3390/msf2021005040 103

Rita Cornamusaz, Francisco Luz, Pedro Brás de Oliveira, Margarida Moncada and Madalena Bettencourt da Câmara
Study of the Phenolic Content and the Antioxidant Capacity of *Rubus idaeus* L. Genotypes within the Development of a National Cultivar
Reprinted from: *Medical Sciences Forum* **2021**, *5*, 41, doi:10.3390/msf2021005041 105

Adinylson Fonseca, Maria Alexandra Bernardo, Maria Fernanda de Mesquita, José Brito and Maria Leonor Silva
Effect of 6% Maltodextrin Intake on Capillary Lactate Concentration in Soccer Players
Reprinted from: *Medical Sciences Forum* **2021**, *5*, 42, doi:10.3390/msf2021005042 107

Lara Costa e Silva, Júlia Teles and Isabel Fragoso
Influence of Maturation on Sports Injuries Profile in Portuguese Youth
Reprinted from: *Medical Sciences Forum* **2021**, *5*, 43, doi:10.3390/msf2021005043 111

Carla F. Rodrigues, Hélder Raposo, Elsa Pegado and Ana I. Fernandes
Coffee in the Workplace: A Social Break or a Performance Enhancer?
Reprinted from: *Medical Sciences Forum* **2021**, *5*, 44, doi:10.3390/msf2021005044 113

Marta Costa, Sara Neves, Joana Carvalho, Sofia Arantes-Oliveira and Sérgio Félix
In Vitro Comparative Study of Microhardness and Flexural Strength of Acrylic Resins Used in Removable Dentures
Reprinted from: *Medical Sciences Forum* **2021**, 5, 45, doi:10.3390/msf2021005045 . . . . **117**

Mafalda Padinha, Cátia Oliveira, Sandra Carlos, Ana Paula Santos, Marta Brito, Carla Adriana Santos and Jorge Fonseca
Long-Term Intestinal Failure and Home Parenteral Nutrition: A Single Center Experience
Reprinted from: *Medical Sciences Forum* **2021**, 5, 46, doi:10.3390/msf2021005046 . . . . **119**

About the Editors

Helena Barroso (Associate Professor) Degree in Pharmaceutical Sciences, Master's in Microbial Molecular Genetics, PhD in Pharmacy (Microbiology). Associate Professor in Health Sciences Institute Egas Moniz, where she teaches since 1998 in the field of Microbiology. Invited Researcher of the Unit for Retroviruses and Associated Infections, Molecular Pathogenesis Center (URIA-CPM) between 2005 and 2013. Researcher from Centro de Investigação Interdisciplinar Egas Moniz (CiiEM) since 2013, being responsible for the research Thematic Area of Microbiology and Public Health. Main areas of interest are HIV infection, bacterial infections and antibiotic resistance. She has been involved in several research projects in these areas. She is the Head of Applied Microbiology Laboratory Egas Moniz since 2010. She authored several scientific papers in indexed international journals and has experience in the supervision of postgraduate students.

Cidália Castro (Assistant Professor) PhD in Advanced Nursing. Master in Nursing. Master in Health Communication. Specialist in Medical-Surgical Nursing in the area of Nursing for the Person in Critical Situation Coordinating Professor of the Nursing Degree Course at the Egas Moniz School of Health. Researcher at the Egas Moniz Interdisciplinary Research Center. Extensive professional experience in the provision of nursing care to persons in critical situations (emergency service and Intensive Care Unit). Published articles in specialized magazines and interacted with collaborators in co-authorship of scientific papers. Jury for masters and doctoral theses in the field of nursing.

Preface to "The 5th International Congress of CiiEM—Reducing inequalities in Health and Society"

Helena Barroso and Cidália Castro

The 5th International Congress of CiiEM (5th IC CiiEM) took place from 16–18 June 2021, as a multidisciplinary scientific online forum focused on Reducing Inequalities in Health and Society. The congress brought together experts from several fields to present their latest findings, experiences and proposals. It included topics like Personalized Health Intervention, Infectious Diseases and Improving Global Health, Decoding the Role of the Environment and Digital Transformation in Health. During three exciting days, 36 invited keynote speakers presented their work, along with several free communications. During the last afternoon, six thematic sessions went on simultaneously, where more than 30 specialists discussed various topics related to specific areas of knowledge. It was a fruitful scientific event, and a model towards a more comprehensive approach to the current and future challenges in health and society.

Statement of Peer Review

In submitting conference proceedings to *Proceedings*, the volume editors of the proceedings certify to the publisher that all papers published in this volume have been subjected to peer review administered by the volume editors. Reviews were conducted by expert referees to the professional and scientific standards expected of a proceedings journal.

- Type of peer review: Double-blind
- Conference submission management system: Wordpress Plugin WP Abstracts Pro v.2.3.0 Abstracts & Manuscripts Submission
- Number of submissions sent for review: 53
- Number of submissions accepted: 47 (11 oral and 36 poster presentations)
- Acceptance rate (number of submissions accepted/number of submissions received): 88.7%
- Average number of reviews per paper: 2
- Total number of reviewers involved: 61
- Any additional information on the review process: The reviewers' comments regarding scientific soundness and formatting of the works were considered by the editors, who were ultimately responsible for guaranteeing the corrections needed and made the final approval / rejection decision. The nominal list of those involved in the evaluation process is included in the acknowledgements.

Acknowledgments

The works submitted to the congress, spanning across several areas of knowledge, were subjected to a thorough double-blind peer-review. We acknowledge the input of the colleagues who contributed to more scientifically sound proceedings.

Board of Editors

Ana Isabel Fernandes
Fernanda Loureiro
Madalena Salema Oom

Renata Ramalho
Sónia Vicente

Board of Reviewers

Aida Duarte
Aida Serra
Alexandra Bernardo
Alexandra M Silva
Alexandra Pinto
Alexandre Quintas Ana Azul
Ana Cristina Vidal Ana Neves
Ana Paula Serro
Ana Vanessa Antunes
André Mariz Almeida
Ângela Pereira
Armando Sena
Carlos Família
Carlos Monteiro Carlos Zagalo Catarina Bernardes Catarina Ramos Cecília Rozan
Cidália Castro
Cláudia Costa
Cristina Soeiro
Deolinda Auxtero
Edite Torres
Eunice Carrilho
Filipa Vicente
Guilhermina Moutinho
Helder Costa
Helena Barroso
Inês Caldeira Fernandes
Isabel M Costa
João Aguiar
João Dias
João Paulo Sousa
Jorge Caldeira
Jorge Cardoso
Jorge Fonseca
José Feliz
José Grillo
Júlio Fernandes
Luisa B Lopes
Leonor Silva
Margarida Ferreira
Miguel Garcia
Nuno Taveira
Patricia C Silva
Paula Oliveira
Paula Pereira
Paulo Maia
Paulo Maurício
Pedro M Pereira
Pedro Oliveira
Perpétua Gomes
Sérgio Félix
Sofia Pinto
Susana Monteiro
Telma Almeida
Teresa Nascimento
Veronique Sena
Vítor Tavares

Helena Barroso, Cidália Castro
Editors

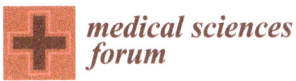

Proceeding Paper

Dispensing of Food Supplements in the Treatment and Prevention of Urinary Tract Infections [†]

Beatriz Setoca and Ana I. Fernandes *

CiiEM, Interdisciplinary Research Center Egas Moniz, Instituto Universitário Egas Moniz, Quinta da Granja, Monte de Caparica, 2829-511 Caparica, Portugal; beatrizdfpsetoca@gmail.com
* Correspondence: aifernandes@egasmoniz.edu.pt; Tel.: +351-212946823
† Presented at the 5th International Congress of CiiEM—Reducing Inequalities in Health and Society, Online, 16–18 June 2021.

Abstract: Urinary tract infections constitute an important public health issue due to recurrence and antibiotic resistance. Currently, antibiotics are the standard therapy but non-antibiotic approaches, such as food supplements, could be beneficial and reduce bacterial resistance. This work aimed at a better understanding of the perception of health professionals involved in dispensing and counselling, in the community pharmacy, regarding the utility of these products as preventive alternatives and therapeutic approaches.

Keywords: food supplements; urinary tract infections; prevention; treatment

1. Introduction

Urinary tract infections (UTI) are one of the most common infections, both in healthcare and in the community setting [1]. Currently, antibiotics (e.g., fosfomycin) are the standard therapy, but the high rates of infection recurrence and antibiotic resistance pose an important public health problem. With that in mind, the management of this pathology using non-antibiotic therapies, such as food supplements (FS), are considered an asset and could reduce resistance. However, the use of FS in the treatment and prevention of UTI is still controversial, since the associated risks and benefits are unknown to many health professionals (HP) [2].

An in-depth study of the scientific evidence available is; therefore, warranted to enable informed dispensing and counselling of these products in community pharmacies. The aim of this study was to evaluate the consumption of FS for the prophylaxis and/or treatment of UTI in Portugal and assess differences of pharmacist's behavior vs non-pharmacists towards their recommendation.

2. Materials and Methods

Sales data (2017 to 2019) of FS indicated in UTI management were obtained from the National Pharmacies Association (ANF), representing about 95% of the national pharmacies. Eighty-five FS were analyzed to identify the alleged bioactive molecules and the labelling of the five top sellers examined, from the perspective of efficacy and safety. To characterize the dispensing and counselling act, in the context of treatment/prevention of UTI, an anonymous online questionnaire (approved by Egas Moniz's Ethics Committee) was applied to HP working in a community pharmacy (inclusion criteria). Besides pattern of dispensing/counselling, preference and the perception of quality, safety and efficacy were also evaluated. The questionnaire was shared on social media, in specific professional groups, and emailed to 200 community pharmacies. Responses (n = 149) were collected between April and October 2020. The study was complemented with a literature review in databases, such as Cochrane Library and PubMed.

3. Results and Discussion

Results show increased (~44%) dispensing of FS for UTI, in pharmacies, from 2017 to 2019, which may suggest either an increasing prevalence of UTI or a higher demand of these products by consumers. The top selling FS are sold as hard gelatin capsules and present a great diversity of alleged bioactives (mainly *Vaccinium macrocarpon*—cranberry, *Arctostaphylos uva-ursi*—bearberry and *Lactobacillus sp.*—probiotics), many of them combined in the same formulation, which potentiates adverse reactions and interactions. Required legal labelling mentions were present in every product; indication of the maximum/ideal duration of consumption and minimum age for intake were lacking. Many products recommended that a HP should be notified in cases of combined use of anticoagulants, antiplatelet agents and in pregnancy, or lactation. Yet, since there are no official recommendations, it is up to the HP to advise, or not, the use of FS in these situation.

Most of the respondents to the questionnaire (n = 149), involved in FS dispensing and counselling, were pharmacists (78%); technicians and assistant technicians account for the remaining professionals. FS for UTI are dispensed frequently (once/twice a week) in the pharmacy, by 42% of the professionals; 92% of these dispensing acts are reported as accompanied by counselling.

Although FS cannot claim the treatment or prevention of disease, a majority of the HP believe that FS are important in UTI, as adjuvants to drug therapy (n = 122), in prevention (n = 93) or even as treatment (n = 59). Although clinical studies and meta-analysis available in literature do not clearly demonstrate the efficacy of the FS in UTI [2], only a minority of the HP (n = 4) believe that they are not important in these infections, due to lack of safety (0.7%) or inefficacy (2%).

An independent question cross-checked perception of quality, efficacy and safety with respect to FS. Again, only 12% of the professionals consider that FS do not attain the minimum requisites; the vast majority of pharmacists consider FS as being safe and of quality. Efficacy is perceived only by a minority (13%) of non-pharmacists; perception of pharmacists is in line with the existing lack of evidence regarding these products, found in the literature. HP in community pharmacies, represented by 91% of pharmacists, 93% of technicians and 83% of assistant technicians, believe that regulation and inspection of FS should be similar to that of medicines. A significant number of pharmacists also consider that publicity (16%) and regulation (11%) of FS should be reviewed, though retaining the status of foods. The need to include FS in the pharmacovigilance system, providing monitoring regarding potential interactions and contraindications, was also mentioned.

The majority of HP (54%) reported not to indicate a specific product (brand) to the consumer. Pharmacists (47%) are those who tend to have a product of election; choice is justified by perception of efficacy previously reported, or confidence in the manufacturer of the FS. The main bioactives indicated were cranberry (59%) and bearberry (14%), coinciding with the consumption data.

In conclusion, though HP in community pharmacies consider FS as a safe and important non-pharmacological approach in the management of UTI, there is agreement with the need for further scientific evidence on safety and efficacy, as well as to bring FS regulation closer to that of medicines.

Funding: This research received no external funding.

Institutional Review Board Statement: The study was conducted according to the guidelines of the Declaration of Helsinki, and approved by the Ethics Committee of Egas Moniz (protocol code 799; date of approval: 19 December 2019).

Informed Consent Statement: Informed consent was obtained from all subjects involved in the study.

Acknowledgments: ANF is acknowledged for providing the FS sales data.

Conflicts of Interest: The authors declare no conflict of interest.

References

1. Medina, M.; Castillo-Pino, E. An introduction to the epidemiology and burden of urinary tract infections. *Ther. Adv. Urol.* **2019**, *11*. [CrossRef] [PubMed]
2. Cai, T.; Tamanini, I.; Kulchavenya, E.; Perepanova, T.; Köves, B.; Wagenlehner, F.M.; Tandogdu, Z.; Bonkat, G.; Bartoletti, R.; Johansen, T.E.B. The role of nutraceuticals and phytotherapy in the management of urinary tract infections: What we need to know? *Arch. Ital. Urol. Androl.* **2017**, *89*, 1–6. [CrossRef] [PubMed]

Proceeding Paper

Cohesiveness of Powdered Co-Amorphous Olanzapine and Impact on Tablet Production †

Nuno F. da Costa [1], João F. Pinto [1] and Ana I. Fernandes [2,*]

1. iMed.ULisboa, Departamento de Farmácia Galénica e Tecnologia Farmacêutica, Faculdade de Farmácia, Universidade de Lisboa, Av. Prof. Gama Pinto, P-1649-003 Lisboa, Portugal; nparferreira@gmail.com (N.F.d.C.); jfpinto@ff.ul.pt (J.F.P.)
2. CiiEM—Interdisciplinary Research Center Egas Moniz, Instituto Universitário Egas Moniz, Monte de Caparica, P-2829-511 Caparica, Portugal
* Correspondence: aifernandes@egasmoniz.edu.pt; Tel.: +351-212-946-823
† Presented at the 5th International Congress of CiiEM—Reducing Inequalities in Health and Society, Online, 16–18 June 2021.

Abstract: The evaluation of the processability of co-amorphous mixtures is of paramount importance since these systems are increasingly used to address the poor solubility presented by most of the drugs in research and development. This work shows that co-amorphous olanzapine powders present higher cohesiveness than their crystalline counterpart and resulted in the production of tablets with a higher tensile strength and a slower release of the drug. As a result, this work demonstrates that despite the solubility advantages of co-amorphous mixtures, consideration should be given to the downstream processing of formulations containing such materials.

Keywords: co-amorphous; cohesiveness; dissolution; olanzapine; tablets; tensile strength

1. Introduction

Co-amorphization of drugs has been extensively described as an adequate approach to overcome the poor bioavailability issues faced by a significant fraction of drug substances (approximately 70%) [1] currently under research and development. Though of paramount importance, assessment of the processability of co-amorphous systems for the manufacture of medicines is still lacking [2]. This work aimed at evaluating the cohesiveness of crystalline vs. co-amorphous olanzapine/saccharin powder mixtures, and the attributes of tablets produced with these materials.

2. Materials and Methods

Olanzapine (OLZ, Rampex Labs, Telangana, India) and saccharin (SAC, Sigma-Aldrich, Steinheim, Germany) were dissolved in dichloromethane (Biochem Chemopharma, Cosne sur Loire, France) and co-amorphized by evaporating the solvent at 45 °C/650 mbar (Buchi Rotavapor, Buchi, Flawil, Switzerland) [3]. Rheological characterization of crystalline physical mixtures of OLZ and SAC and the co-amorphous system was carried out in a TA.XT Plus Texture Analyzer fitted with a powder flow accessory (Stable Micro Systems, Surrey, United Kingdom). The cohesion index was determined as the ratio between the work required to move the blade upwards (75 mm/s) and the weight of the sample (30 g). To produce tablets, OLZ (30%), either as a crystalline mixture with SAC (18%) or in the co-amorphous system, was blended with anhydrous dibasic calcium phosphate (27%, Budenheim, Budenheim, Germany), microcrystalline cellulose (20%, FMC Corp., Cork, Ireland) and povidone (5%, BASF, Ludwigshafen, Germany). Blended samples (66.5 mg manually weighted) were used to fill the compression die (5 mm diameter, Lloyd Instruments, Largo, FL, USA) and compressed (90 MPa at a constant speed of 10 mm/min). Tablets were characterized based on tensile strength (TA.XT Plus fitted with a cylinder probe, Stable Micro Systems, Surrey, United Kingdom), disintegration time (demineralized water, 37 ± 2 °C, Erweka, Heusenstamm, Germany) and dissolution testing using the paddle method (100 rpm, 37 ± 2 °C, Sotax, Aesch, Switzerland) and pH 6.8 phosphate buffer (300 mL) as the dissolution medium.

3. Results and Discussion

Co-amorphization of OLZ and SAC was previously described as a useful method to enhance the water solubility and dissolution rate of OLZ [3]. However, co-amorphization of OLZ resulted in the production of a powdered system presenting a higher cohesion index (25.2 ± 1.2) than its crystalline counterpart (12.7 ± 0.4). The higher cohesiveness of co-amorphous OLZ may be explained by the increased mobility of its molecules at the surface of the particles, thus impacting negatively on the flow. As a consequence of the poor flowability of the co-amorphous OLZ, an unacceptable mass and content uniformity are expected, negatively impacting on the therapeutic effectiveness of the dosage form and rendering batches uncompliant with pharmacopoeia standards.

Tableting of blends containing co-amorphous OLZ resulted in the preparation of compacts with a higher tensile strength (1.97 ± 0.01 MPa) than those produced with the physical mixture of crystalline OLZ and SAC (1.01 ± 0.05 MPa). The higher tensile strength of compacts made with a co-amorphous OLZ probably relates to the higher cohesiveness of co-amorphous OLZ, whose particles also seem to be more elastic and plastic than the crystalline equivalents. Moreover, during compaction, the temperature of the powder bed increased and may have approached, or even exceeded, the glass transition temperature of the co-amorphous OLZ (57 °C), favoring the rubbery state of the system. Thus, the disintegration time of tablets made of co-amorphous OLZ was significantly higher (420.0 ± 87.2 s) than that of tablets produced with crystalline OLZ/SAC (48.7 ± 4.5 s). This difference is also supported by the mechanism of disintegration observed: while for crystalline OLZ/SAC tablets, compacts disintegrated upon contact with water, tablets made of co-amorphous OLZ slowly and continuously eroded. As a consequence, a slower release of OLZ from tablets made of co-amorphous OLZ was particularly relevant at the beginning of the dissolution test (Figure 1) carried out under sink conditions.

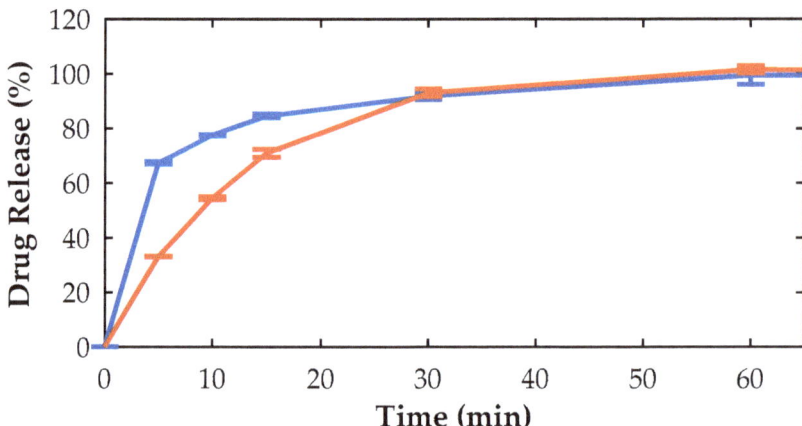

Figure 1. Dissolution profile of tablets produced from physical mixtures of crystalline (blue) and co-amorphous (orange) OLZ/SAC.

In view of the results, downstream processing of formulations containing co-amorphous materials should be given consideration, since they present different bulk flow properties which impact on the quality of the product.

Informed Consent Statement: Not applicable.

Data Availability Statement: Not applicable.

Acknowledgments: The authors acknowledge Fundação para a Ciência e a Tecnologia, Lisbon, Portugal, for providing financial support to this work (PTDC/CTM-BIO/3946/2014 and SFRH/BD/137080/2018).

Conflicts of Interest: The authors declare no conflict of interest.

References

1. Da Costa, N.F.; Pinto, J.F.; Fernandes, A.I. Co-amorphization of olanzapine for solubility enhancement. *Ann. Med.* **2019**, *51*, 87. [CrossRef]
2. Lenz, E.; Jensen, K.T.; Blaabjerg, L.I.; Knop, K.; Grohganz, H.; Löbmann, K.; Rades, T.; Kleinebudde, P. Solid-state properties and dissolution behaviour of tablets containing co-amorphous indomethacin–arginine. *Eur. J. Pharm. Biopharm.* **2015**, *96*, 44–52. [CrossRef] [PubMed]
3. Da Costa, N.F.; Fernandes, A.I.; Pinto, J.F. Measurement of the amorphous fraction of olanzapine incorporated in a co-amorphous formulation. *Int. J. Pharm.* **2020**, *588*, 119716. [CrossRef] [PubMed]

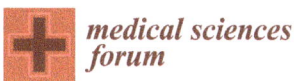

Proceeding Paper

Can Fused Deposition Modelling Enable the Manufacture of Uniform and Precise Dose Tablets? †

Joana Macedo [1,*], **Valérie Vanhoorne** [2], **Chris Vervaet** [2] **and João F. Pinto** [1,*]

1. iMed.ULisboa, Faculdade de Farmácia, Universidade de Lisboa, 1649-003 Lisboa, Portugal
2. Laboratory of Pharmaceutical Technology, Ghent University, 9000 Ghent, Belgium; Valerie.Vanhoorne@ugent.be (V.V.); Chris.Vervaet@ugent.be (C.V.)
* Correspondence: joana.macedo@ff.ulisboa.pt (J.M.); jfpinto@ff.ulisboa.pt (J.F.P.); Tel.: +351-217-946-434 (J.F.P.)
† Presented at the 5th International Congress of CiiEM—Reducing Inequalities in Health and Society, Online, 16–18 June 2021.

Abstract: The consistency of a printer to manufacture tablets in a uniform and precise fashion is an important element when considering fused deposition modelling. Blends of polymer [poly(vinyl alcohol)] and drug (paracetamol) in different ratios were considered to evaluate the mass, drug content, dissolution performance, and thermal properties of tablets. Relative standard deviations below 5%, for most of the properties considered in the study, demonstrated the high uniformity between tablets within a batch and between batches. Overall, the study confirmed the ability of the technology to manufacture tablets in a reproducible way based on the selected properties.

Keywords: 3D printing; fused deposition modelling; poly(vinyl alcohol); paracetamol; solid dosage

1. Introduction

Compounding has been used to obtain a medicine tailored to the specific needs of patients. However, poor compounding practices can result in patient injury and, eventually, death, due to contamination of the medicine or to potency errors [1]. The use of 3D printing has the ability to change the current approach on individualization of medicines. The aim of the present work was to evaluate how consistent fused deposition modelling (FDM) 3D printing can be in the manufacture of tablets based on different critical quality attributes (CQAs: mass, drug content, drug release, and thermal properties) when different blends of poly(vinyl alcohol) (PVA) and paracetamol (PAR) were applied.

2. Materials and Methods

2.1. Preparation of Filaments by Hot-Melt Extrusion (HME) and Tablets by FDM 3D Printing

To prepare feedstock material for FDM 3D printing, mixtures of PVA:PAR (90:10, 70:30, and 50:50 w/w) were extruded (at 0.3 kg/h, 1.75 mm die) in a co-rotating (100 rpm), fully intermeshing twin-screw extruder (Prism Eurolab 16, Thermo Fisher, Karlsruhe, Germany). Thereafter, filaments were fed to a MakerBot Replicator 2X Experimental 3D Printer (MakerBot, Brooklyn, USA), enabling the printing of 30 tablets (10 mm φ and 4 mm thick) of each blend in individual runs (intra-batch variability). To assess inter-batch variability, 2 batches were printed from each blend. The temperature was set at 180, 165, and 150 °C for PVA:PAR 90:10, 70:30 and 50:50, respectively, allowing constant flow out of the nozzle.

2.2. Characterization of Tablets

The mass of each tablet was determined immediately after manufacture. The drug content of tablets (n = 3) was checked in phosphate buffer pH 6.8 (spectrophotometer, λ = 244 nm, UV-1650PC, Shimadzu, Shimadzu Benelux, Antwerp, Belgium). The drug released from tablets was determined by dissolution tests (n = 3, phosphate buffer pH 6.8,

37.0 ± 0.5 °C, paddles at 100 rpm, VK 7010, Vankel Industries, Edison, NJ, USA) in samples collected at pre-set time points. The mean dissolution time enabled the comparison between different profiles. Thermal analysis (*n* = 2) was performed by differential calorimetry (Q2000, TA Instruments, Leatherhead, UK) at 10 °C/min on samples (~5 mg) in T_{zero} pans.

3. Results and Discussion

Results of the CQAs (Table 1) have shown that the Pharmacopoeia requirements for mass uniformity were reached for all formulations, with a variability intra-batch below 0.8%. Nevertheless, a difference of about 10 mg on the average mass was detected between batches of different blends. In this regard, the variation of the filament's diameter plays a major role in printing, especially on the mass deviation of the printed tablet [2]. Printed tablets presented a drug content between 95.5% and 100.6% of the expected value for paracetamol, reflecting the high precision of the process. Moreover, intra- and inter-batch variability was low, as required for the desired therapeutical effect on the patient.

Table 1. Critical quality attributes (CQA) of 3D printed tablets from different batches made of PVA:PAR.

CQA (Average ± Relative Standard Deviation)	Batch	PVA:PAR (% *w/w*)		
		90:10	70:30	50:50
Mass (mg ± %)	1	395.5 ± 0.5	383.5 ± 0.7	375.4 ± 0.5
	2	402.9 ± 0.4	393.5 ± 0.7	385.1 ± 0.8
Drug Content (mg ± %)	1	37.8 ± 1.0	114.0 ± 0.9	183.8 ± 0.2
	2	40.5 ± 1.5	117.0 ± 0.2	183.9 ± 0.9
Mean Dissolution Time (min ± %)	1	47.2 ± 0.9	27.1 ± 0.7	31.7 ± 10.4
	2	46.5 ± 6.1	30.4 ± 0.5	32.0 ± 6.6
ΔC_p [(J/(g·°C)) ± %]	1	0.73 ± 3.7	0.48 ± 4.9	0.33 ± 3.7
	2	0.70 ± 1.4	0.49 ± 0.7	0.31 ± 2.3
$\Delta H_{melting}$ [(J/g) ± %]	1	Not detected	3.48 ± 9.6	69.63 ± 2.5
	2	Not detected	3.68 ± 16.7	67.37 ± 4.2

Considering that FDM is a thermal process, and the dissolution behaviour can be influenced by the state of the solid drug, it was important to confirm whether the printed tablets have kept the value of the enthalpy of either amorphous or crystalline forms of PAR across manufacture. The melting event of tablets have shown that, at low PAR content, full conversion to the amorphous form was obtained, while at 50% PAR the drug remained mostly in the crystalline form, possibly due to the low temperature used, below the melting of the drug. Results have shown a consistent average of the heat capacity (ΔC_p) and enthalpy ($\Delta H_{melting}$) changes between batches and a relative standard deviation below 5% within the batches. However, the enthalpy of the melting event for tablets with 30% PAR showed high deviations within a batch, possibly due to the low crystalline fraction of PAR close to the sensitivity of the technique.

Overall, the study has proved the ability of FDM 3D printing to produce batches of tablets with low intra- and inter-batch variability, regardless the formulation considered.

Acknowledgments: Fundação para a Ciência e a Tecnologia, Lisboa, Portugal, is acknowledged for funding under grants SFRH/BD/125212/2016 and PTDC/CTM CTM/30949/2017 (Lisboa 010145 Feder 030949).

Conflicts of Interest: The authors declare no conflict of interest.

References

1. Gudeman, J.; Jozwiakowski, M.; Chollet, J.; Randell, M. Potential risks of pharmacy compounding. *Drugs R D* **2013**, *13*, 1–8. [CrossRef] [PubMed]
2. Ponsar, H.; Wiedey, R.; Quodbach, J. Hot-melt extrusion process fluctuations and their impact on critical quality attributes of filaments and 3d-printed dosage forms. *Pharmaceutics* **2020**, *12*, 511. [CrossRef] [PubMed]

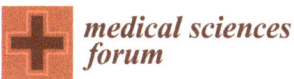

Proceeding Paper

Nutraceuticals for Smart Aging and Potential Drug Interactions [†]

Maria D. Auxtero, Mário Abade, Susana Chalante, Bianca Silva and Ana I. Fernandes *

CiiEM, Interdisciplinary Research Center Egas Moniz, Instituto Universitário Egas Moniz, Quinta da Granja, Monte de Caparica, 2829-511 Caparica, Portugal; mauxtero@egasmoniz.edu.pt (M.D.A.); mario.abade91@gmail.com (M.A.); susanachalante1@sapo.pt (S.C.); biancacosilva@gmail.com (B.S.)
* Correspondence: aifernandes@egasmoniz.edu.pt; Tel.: +351-21-294-6823
† Presented at the 5th International Congress of CiiEM—Reducing Inequalities in Health and Society, Online, 16–18 June 2021.

Abstract: The use of nutraceuticals as cognitive enhancers is on the rise and may be especially problematic in polymedicated older patients. The potential of interaction of these products with drugs commonly prescribed to this age group is evaluated in this work, by identification of mutual targets (enzymes, transporters and receptors).

Keywords: nutraceuticals; aging; cognitive enhancement; drug interactions

1. Introduction

Nutraceuticals are increasingly being used in the management of age-related cognitive disorders [1,2] due to the combination of neuroprotection and/or neurotransmission. However, these products are not exempt from adverse effects and pharmacological interactions, presenting a special risk in older, multimorbid and polymedicated individuals. Understanding pharmacokinetic (PK) and pharmacodynamic (PD) interactions allows anticipation of adverse drug reactions and therapeutic failure.

This study reviews the mechanism of action and interactions between bioactive compounds used for cognitive enhancement and representative drugs, of ten different pharmacotherapeutic classes, usually prescribed to older patients.

2. Materials and Methods

The composition of 25 common nutraceuticals used for cognitive enhancement of adults over 50 years was evaluated. Four bioactive molecules (bacoside A (BA), salidroside (SD), deanol (DE) and homotaurine (HT)) and two plant extracts (*Bacopa monnieri* (BM) and *Rodhiola rosea* (RR)) were selected for further characterization. Propranolol (Pr), alprazolam (Al), sertraline (Se), metformin (Mt), diclofenac (Di), atorvastatin (At), tadalafil (Ta), memantine (Me), piracetam (Pi) and clopidogrel (Cl) were the drugs selected. A full PK/PD profile was obtained for each drug, focusing on the role of multiple enzymes, transporters and receptors, and identifying common targets of the bioactive molecules, as a measure of potential drug/nutraceutical interaction. Databases such as Cochrane Library, Science Direct, PubMed, MedlinePlus, WebMD and Drug Bank were consulted.

3. Results and Discussion

HT is the less problematic of the bioactives studied since it only interacts with NMDA receptor, as an antagonist. Both RR and BA (bioactive of BM) show inhibitory effects on monoamine oxidase A and B (MAO A and B). Hence, nutraceuticals containing any of the two bioactives (and tyramine rich food) should be avoided whenever therapeutics include selective serotonin reuptake inhibitors (e.g., Se, a MAO substrate) and blood pressure medication (e.g., Pr, a MAO A inhibitor). P-glycoprotein (P-gp) is a membrane efflux transporter, influencing oral bioavailability of its substrates, such as Pr, Se, Di, At, Ta and Cl. Since P-gp is inhibited by BM and SD, the concomitant use of those drugs may greatly increase their oral bioavailability. Similar to RR and BA, DE showed inhibitory capacity for several cytochrome P450 enzymes, whereas SD proved to be an inducer (Table 1). CYP3A4 is responsible for the metabolism of 70% of the drugs considered and it is inhibited by BA and RR, resulting in decreased plasma clearance of those drugs and increased risk of toxicity. It is of the utmost relevance to fully understand these interactions, in order to prevent side effects, especially with 'High-Alert Medications' (HAM) (60% of those studied) and narrow therapeutic index drugs.

Table 1. Targets of potential interactions between drugs and bioactive molecules (or plant extracts).

Drug	Enzyme (E)/Transporter (T)/Receptor (R)										
	CYP						MAO		P-gp	MRP1	NMDA
	1A2	3A4	2C9	2B6	2D6	2C19	A	B			
Al ▲	-	S BA * RR *	S BA * RR * SD *	-	-	-	-	-	-	-	-
At ▲	-	S BA * RR *	↓BA * RR * SD •	↑SD **	↓DE *	↓BA * DE *	-	-	S↓ BM * SD *	S SD *	-
Cl ▲	S BA * RR * SD • DE *	S BA * RR *	S↓BA * RR * D •	S↓SD •	-	S BA * DE *	-	-	S BM * SD *	-	-
Di ▲	S BA * RR * SD • DE *	S↓BA * RR *	S↓BA * RR * SD •	S SD •	-	S BA * DE *	-	-	↑BM * SD *	↓SD *	-
Me	-	-	-	↓SD •	-	↓BA * DE *	-	-	-	-	AN HT ■
Mt ▲/Pi	-	-	-	-	-	-	-	-	-	-	-
Pr ▲	S BA *RR * SD • DE *	S BA * RR *	-	-	S↓DE *	S BA * DE *	↓BA * RR *	-	S BM * SD *	-	-
Se	-	S BA * RR *	↓BA * RR * SD •	S↓SD •	S↓DE *	S↓BA * DE *	S BA * RR *	S BA * RR *	S↓BM * SD *	-	-
Ta	-	S BA * RR *	-	-	-	-	-	-	S BM * SD *	-	-

S: drug is substrate of E, T or R; ↓: drug is inhibitor of E, T or R; ↑: drug is inducer of E, T or R; AN: drug is antagonist of R; * inhibitor of E, T or R; • inducer of E, T or R; ■ R antagonist; ▲ HAM.

Bioactives of botanical origin are more likely to lead to interaction, as expressed by the higher number of mutual targets affected (up to eight for RR/SD with Di). BA/BM inhibit four main CYP enzymes (2C19, 2C9, 1A2 and 3A4), P-gP and MAO (A/B), thus potentially increasing plasma levels of 70% of the drugs considered (Pr, Al, Se, Di, At, Me, Ta and Cl). RR/BA interact with MAO inhibitors, CYP2C9 substrates and serotonin reuptake inhibitors.

Results confirm that the co-administration of nutraceuticals and drugs can alter PK/PD parameters, resulting in side effects or therapeutic failure. Systematic monitoring of the addition of such products, often erroneously mistaken as medicines, to the therapeutic regimen of polymedicated older patients is especially important.

Data Availability Statement: Not applicable.

Conflicts of Interest: The authors declare no conflict of interest.

References

1. Sut, S.; Baldan, V.; Faggian, M.; Peron, G.; Dall Acqua, S. Nutraceuticals, A New Challenge for Medicinal Chemistry. *Curr. Med. Chem.* **2016**, *23*, 3198–3223. [CrossRef] [PubMed]
2. Wightman, E.L. Potential benefits of phytochemicals against Alzheimer's disease. *Proc. Nutr. Soc.* **2017**, *76*, 106–112. [CrossRef]

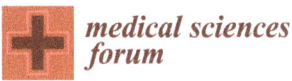

Proceeding Paper

The Profile of People with Parkinson's Disease Included in Community Boxing Exercise Programs †

Josefa Domingos [1,2], Tamine Capato [1,3] and Catarina Godinho [2,*]

1. Department of Neurology, Center of Expertise for Parkinson and Movement Disorders, Donders Institute for Brain, Cognition and Behaviour, Radboud University Medical Center, P.O. Box 9101, 6500 HB Nijmegen, The Netherlands; domingosjosefa@gmail.com (J.D.); taminec@usp.br (T.C.)
2. Grupo de Patologia Médica, Nutrição e Exercício Clínico (PaMNEC) do Centro de Investigação Interdisciplinar Egas Moniz (CiiEM), 2829-511 Caparica, Almada, Portugal
3. Movement Disorders Center, Department of Neurology, University of São Paulo, São Paulo 05403-000, Brazil
* Correspondence: cgodinho@egasmoniz.edu.pt
† Presented at the 5th International Congress of CiiEM—Reducing Inequalities in Health and Society, Online, 16–18 June 2021.

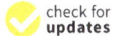

Citation: Domingos, J.; Capato, T.; Godinho, C. The Profile of People with Parkinson's Disease Included in Community Boxing Exercise Programs. *Med. Sci. Forum* **2021**, *5*, 5. https://doi.org/10.3390/msf2021005005

Academic Editors: Helena Barroso and Cidália Castro

Published: 10 July 2021

Publisher's Note: MDPI stays neutral with regard to jurisdictional claims in published maps and institutional affiliations.

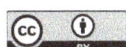

Copyright: © 2021 by the authors. Licensee MDPI, Basel, Switzerland. This article is an open access article distributed under the terms and conditions of the Creative Commons Attribution (CC BY) license (https://creativecommons.org/licenses/by/4.0/).

Abstract: Exercise is widely recommended for people with Parkinson (PD). Boxing is a popular mode of training. However, including individuals with less favorable profiles may have a negative impact on participation. We performed a systematic review to study the patient characteristics that were included in boxing exercise programs research and reflect on the possible inclusion criteria that professionals can use for boxing exercise programs. Indications for the best profiles were limited due to the small number of studies. Boxing programs should include people with the diagnosis of PD in earlier stages, independently ambulatory, and without current severe musculoskeletal or cardiovascular conditions.

Keywords: Parkinson's disease; community exercise; boxing; profiles

1. Introduction

Growing evidence underscores the benefit of exercise programs in individuals with Parkinson PD as a long-term cost-effective and accessible care for ongoing exercise. Several types of community programs are being used [1–3]. Boxing is one of the most popular programs. However, including individuals with less favorable profiles may have a negative impact on the participation [4]. We performed a systematic review to study the patient characteristics that were included in boxing exercise programs and reflection on what type of patients should participate.

2. Materials and Methods

We reviewed the clinical characteristics of the people with PD included in boxing exercise programs. We performed a systematic literature in the databases PubMed, Medline, and the Cochrane library using the following keywords: "Parkinson disease" AND "boxing". We included all studies regarding exercise boxing programs with people diagnosed with PD.

3. Results and Discussion

Three studies were found. Of these, two were both led by Combs. Several inclusion criteria in research studies were identified (Table 1).

Table 1. Summary of characteristics of participants in studies regarding community-based boxing programs Parkinson's disease.

Study & Study Design	Average Age (years)	Time since Diagnosis (months)	Hoehn & Yahr Score	Other Inclusion Criteria
Combs, 2011 [1] Case Series N = 6 M: 6, F: 0	60.17 years (10.26)	28.67 (24.34)	2.17 (1.33)	(1) Complete informed consent form; (2) At least 21 years; (3) Able to ambulate; (4) Able to follow 3-step verbal commands; (5) Self-transportation; (6) No other preexisting neurological conditions other than PD; (7) No musculoskeletal or cardiovascular conditions; (8) Brain surgery or deep brain stimulator; (9) Current pregnancy.
Combs, 2013 [2] RCT n = 31 (Intervention = 17, Control = 14) M: 21 F: 10	Boxing 68.0 years (31.0) Exercise 66.5 years (28.0)	Boxing group 41.5 (182.0) Control group 50.0 (99.0)	Boxing group 2.0 (3.0) Control group 2.0 (3.0)	Similar to previuos study (same authors).
Domingos, 2019 [3] Acceptability	Not reported	Not reported	Not reported	(1) Complete informed consent form; (2) Accept supported by a volunteer if at risk of falls according to screening tests.

RCT = Randomised controlled trial; M, male; F, female. The most favourable characteristics for patients to be included in boxing programs may include younger aged participants with shorter disease duration and in earlier stages of the disease. Exclusion due to cognitive impairment was not reported in neither of the studies.

Institutional Review Board Statement: The study was conducted according to the guidelines of the Declaration of Helsinki.

Informed Consent Statement: Not applicable.

Data Availability Statement: Not applicable.

Conflicts of Interest: The authors declare no conflict of interest.

References

1. Combs, S.A.; Diehl, M.D.; Staples, W.H.; Conn, L.; Davis, K.; Lewis, N.; Schaneman, K. Boxing training for patients with Parkinson disease: A case series. *Phys. Ther.* **2011**, *91*, 132–142. [CrossRef] [PubMed]
2. Combs, S.A.; Diehl, M.D.; Chrzastowski, C.; Didrick, N.; McCoin, B.; Mox, N.; Staples, W.H.; Wayman, J. Community-based group exercise for persons with Parkinson disease: A randomized controlled trial. *NRE* **2013**, *32*, 117–124. [CrossRef] [PubMed]
3. Domingos, J.; Radder, D.; Riggare, S.; Godinho, G.; Dean, J.; Graziano, M.; Vries, N.M.; Ferreira, J.; Bloem, B. Implementation of a Community-Based Exercise Program for Parkinson Patients: Using Boxing as an Example. *JPD* **2019**, *9*, 615–623. [CrossRef] [PubMed]
4. Domingos, J.; Dean, J.; Godinho, C.; Melo, F. Proliferation of community exercise programs with limited evidence and expertise: Safety implications. *Mov. Disord.* **2018**, *33*, 1365–1366. [CrossRef] [PubMed]

Proceeding Paper

Assessment of Hyposalivation, Xerostomia, and Oral Health-Related Quality of Life in Polymedicated Patients †

João Gato Marques [1,*], Cecília Rozan [1], Luís Proença [1,2], André Peixoto [1] and Cristina Manso [1,2]

1. Instituto Universitário Egas Moniz, Campus Universitário, 2829-511 Caparica, Portugal; ceciliarozan@gmail.com (C.R.); lproenca@egasmoniz.edu.pt (L.P.); andrec.peixoto@gmail.com (A.P.); mansocristina@gmail.com (C.M.)
2. Centro de Investigação Interdisciplinar Egas Moniz, 2829-511 Caparica, Portugal
* Correspondence: jgato1997@gmail.com
† Presented at the 5th International Congress of CiiEM—Reducing Inequalities in Health and Society, Online, 16–18 June 2021.

Abstract: To investigate the self-reported impact of hyposalivation/xerostomia on Oral Health-Related Quality of Life (OHRQoL) reported by polymedicated patients and evaluate the association between hyposalivation/xerostomia and OHRQoL. A cross-sectional observational study was performed on 40 polymedicated patients selected from the Clínica Dentária Egas Moniz. The subjects signed a consent form, answered a questionnaire to assess xerostomia via the *Summated Xerostomia Inventory* (SXI-PL) and *The Portuguese short version of the Oral Health Impact Profile Questionnaire* (OHIP-14sp), and underwent sialometry evaluation. Patients with hyposalivation showed higher scores of SXI-PL (8.60 ± 2.56) and OHIP-14sp (16.0 ± 15.8). These findings suggest an association between hyposalivation and SXI-PL and OHIP-14sp scores ($p < 0.05$).

Keywords: hyposalivation; xerostomia; oral health-related quality of life; polymedication

1. Introduction

Saliva is a biochemically complex fluid containing proteins and various glycoproteins, lipids, electrolytes, and buffers, which all play a vital role in oral health. It preserves dentition, inhibits the growth of microorganisms, lubricates and protects the oral mucosa from trauma, and facilitates mastication, deglutition, and speech. Hyposalivation and xerostomia are the most common symptoms associated with polymedication. Consequently, the oral signs and symptoms of hyposalivation and xerostomia extend far beyond those of simple dryness, with a negative impact on patients' quality of life [1]. The aim of this study was to assess the prevalence of hyposalivation and xerostomia in polymedicated patients and their impact on Oral Health-Related Quality of Life (OHRQoL).

2. Materials and Methods

We performed a cross-sectional observational study. We selected 40 polymedicated patients, who were regularly administered at least two of the following medications: anticonvulsants, antidepressants, oral hypoglycemics, antihypertensives, and H1 antihistamines, from the Clínica Dentária Egas Moniz. The study was approved by the Egas Moniz Ethical Committee. The subjects signed a consent form and answered a questionnaire to assess Summated Xerostomia Inventory (SXI-PL) and The Portuguese short version of the Oral Health Impact Profile Questionnaire (OHIP-14sp) and underwent sialometry evaluation to assess unstimulated (USFR) and stimulated (SSFR) salivary flow rates. Hyposalivation was diagnosed for USFR <0.1 mL/min and/or SSFR <0.7 mL/min. A statistical analysis was performed using the software IBM SPSS® Statistics, v.25. Spearman's correlation coefficient was used to analyze the association of the SXI-PL and OHIP-14sp scores with salivary flow rates.

3. Results and Discussion

The prevalence of hyposalivation was 50% in our population. The overall SXI-PL scores ranged from 5 to 15 with a mean of 7.85 (± 2.37). The mean score of SXI-PL was higher in patients with hyposalivation (8.60 ± 2.56). The results demonstrate a statistically significant correlation between SXI-PL scores and hyposalivation (p = 0.0195) (Table 1). The symptom that indicated higher severity of xerostomia was "My mouth feels dry" (2.20 ± 0.70) (Figure 1a).

Table 1. Discriminant validity of Summated Xerostomia Inventory (SXI-PL) and The Portuguese short version of the Oral Health Impact Profile Questionnaire (OHIP-14sp) mean scores for assessing salivary flow conditions.

	Hyposalivation	Normal	Total	p-Value [1]
SXI-PL	8.60 ± 2.56	7.10 ± 1.94	7.85 ± 2.37	0.0195
OHIP-14sp	16.0 ± 15.8	7.0 ± 7.4	11.50 ± 12.98	0.0425

[1] A significance level of 0.05 was considered statistically significant.

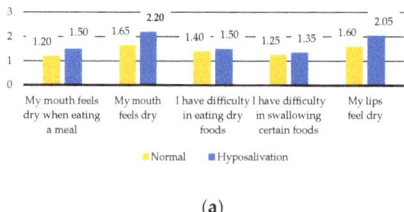 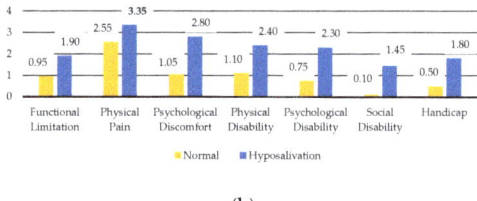

(a) (b)

Figure 1. (a) Distribution of the mean scores of SXI-PL symptoms for different salivary flow condition; (b) distribution of the mean scores of OHIP-14sp dimensions for different salivary flow condition.

The overall OHIP-14sp scores ranged from 0 to 51, with a mean of 11.50 (± 12.98). The mean score of OHIP-14sp was higher in patients with hyposalivation (16.0 ± 15.8). The results demonstrate a statistically significant correlation between OHIP-14sp scores and hyposalivation (p = 0.0425) (Table 1). The dimension of OHIP-14sp with higher impact was "Physical Pain" (3.35 ± 2.81) (Figure 1b).

Munõz et al. determined that xerostomia was prevalent in 55.9% of an elderly population with hyposalivation in Chile [1]. Putten et al. reported that the most severe symptom of xerostomia in a Dutch population was "My mouth feels dry" (1.8 points) [2]. Smidt et al. found an association between hyposalivation and xerostomia in Copenhagen inhabitants (p < 0.001) [3].

Ikebe et al. performed a study of hyposalivation and its impact on OHRQoL in an elderly Japanese population. The results demonstrated that subjects with hyposalivation reported higher OHIP-14 scores (14.6 ± 8.3) and showed a higher impact on the "Physical Pain" dimension (1.5 points). An association between hyposalivation and OHIP-14 was found (p = 0.011) [4].

In the present study, an association between hyposalivation and xerostomia was found in polymedicated patients, which has a negative impact on oral health-related quality of life.

Conflicts of Interest: The authors declare no conflict of interest.

References

1. Munõz, C.; Martínez, A.; Flores, M.; Catalán, A. Relationship between Xerostomia and Hyposalivation in Senior Chilean People. *Rev. Clin. Periodoncia Implantol. Rehabil. Oral* **2019**, *12*, 123–126. [CrossRef]
2. Putten, G.J.; Brand, H.S.; Schols, J.M.; Baat, C. The diagnostic suitability of a xerostomia questionnaire and the association between xerostomia, hyposalivation and medication use in a group of nursing home residents. *Clin. Oral Investig.* **2011**, *15*, 185–192. [CrossRef] [PubMed]

3. Smidt, D.; Torpet, L.A.; Nauntofte, B.; Heegaard, K.M.; Pedersen, A.M. Associations between oral and ocular dryness, labial and whole salivary flow rates, systemic diseases and medications in a sample of older people. *Community Dent. Oral Epidemiol.* **2011**, *39*, 276–288. [CrossRef] [PubMed]
4. Ikebe, K.; Matsuda, K.; Morii, K.; Wada, M.; Hazeyama, T.; Nokubi, T.; Ettinger, R.L. Impact of dry mouth and hyposalivation on oral health-related quality of life of elderly Japanese. *Oral Surg. Oral Med. Oral Pathol. Oral Radiol. Endod.* **2007**, *103*, 216–222. [CrossRef] [PubMed]

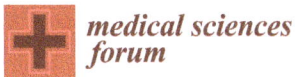

Proceeding Paper

Evaluation of the Cytotoxic Potential of Adhesives, with Two on the Market: Scotchbond Universal and Optibond Solo Plus, and an Adhesive in the Experimental Phase: T1 [†]

Sofia Santos [1], Paulo Mascarenhas [1], Susana Bandarra [1], Ana Clara Ribeiro [1], Paulo Maurício [2] and Isabel Barahona [1,*]

1. Laboratório de Biologia Molecular, Centro de Investigação Interdisciplinar Egas Moniz (CiiEM), Instituto Universitário Egas Moniz (IUEM), 2829-511 Caparica, Portugal; sosantos@gmail.com (S.S.); pmascarenhas@egasmoniz.edu.pt (P.M.); sbandarra@egasmoniz.edu.pt (S.B.); acribeiro@egasmoniz.edu.pt (A.C.R.)
2. Clínica Dentária Egas Moniz, Instituto Universitário Egas Moniz (IUEM), 2829-511 Caparica, Portugal; dmauricio@netcabo.pt
* Correspondence: ibarahona@egasmoniz.edu.pt
† Presented at the 5th International Congress of CiiEM—Reducing Inequalities in Health and Society, Online, 16–18 June 2021.

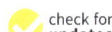

Abstract: In vitro studies evaluating the cytotoxic potential of substances released from dental adhesives are lacking. The purpose of this study was to compare the cytotoxicity of the extracts of dental adhesives Scotchbond Universal and Optibond Solo Plus, and an adhesive in the experimental phase: T1. 3T3 mouse fibroblast cells and MG-63 osteoblast-like cells from human osteosarcoma were exposed for 24 h to serial extract dilutions. Cytotoxicity was determined using an MTT assay. For both cell lines, the cytotoxicity order obtained, of the unfiltered adhesive extracts, was T1 (less cytotoxic) < Optibond Solo Plus < Scotchbond Universal (most cytotoxic).

Keywords: dental adhesives; cytotoxicity; MTT Assay; cell viability

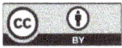

1. Introduction

Dental adhesives are widely used in dentistry. They serve as intermediate agents, which presupposes a direct and lasting contact with the dental structure. Studies show that after the application of adhesive agents to the already conditioned dentin, some residual monomers, from degradation or incomplete polymerization process, as well as other components of the adhesive systems, can penetrate and diffuse through the dentinal tubules and consequently reach the dental pulp, triggering inflammatory processes [1]. Resin monomers traditionally present in the composition of adhesive systems have a certain degree of cytotoxicity [2,3]. New adhesives are being produced permanently with better adhesive properties and easier application, but for long lasting restoration, they also have to be biocompatible. The purpose of this investigation was to evaluate the cytotoxic potential of three types of adhesives, the Scotchbond Universal (two-step self-etch universal generation adhesive), Optibond Solo Plus (two-step Etch-Rinse or one-step self-etch 5th generation adhesive), and a new adhesive in the experimental phase, T1.

2. Materials and Methods

The adhesives were brushed in petri dishes, polymerized, immersed in culture medium, and incubated for 24 h for extracts preparation. The cytotoxicity experiments were performed in mouse embryo fibroblast cells (NIH/3T3; ATCC CRL-1658) and human osteoblast-like cells from osteosarcoma (MG-63; ATCC CRL-1427) exposed to different extracts dilutions. For cytotoxic evaluation, 1×10^4 cells per well, from passages 8 to 12, were seeded in 96-well plates (eight replicates) and incubated at 37 °C for 24 h under a humidified atmosphere of 5% CO_2. After proliferation, the growth medium was removed and replaced with 200 μL per well of undiluted extracts or serial dilutions of each adhesive extract (up to 1:50). Unexposed control cells were incubated with growth medium only. MTT assays were performed as previously described [4]. After 24 h of incubation with the potentially toxic compounds, we measured the formazan crystals formed at 595 nm absorbance and the unexposed control cells were considered to indicate 100% cell viability. A minimum of three independent assays were performed. Statistical analysis was performed through an analysis of variance (ANOVA) followed by Tukey's HSD multiple comparison test.

3. Results and Discussion

The results obtained for the three adhesives are displayed in Figure 1, as cellular viability after exposure to different adhesive extract concentrations. For 3T3 fibroblasts, the cytotoxicity order obtained of the unfiltered adhesive extracts was T1 (less cytotoxic) < Optibond Solo Plus < Scotchbond Universal (most cytotoxic).

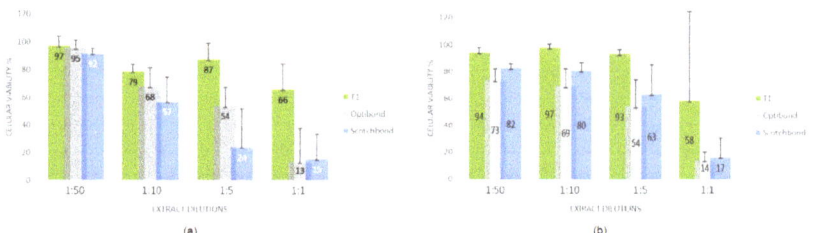

Figure 1. Cytotoxicity of unfiltered (**a**) and filtered (**b**) adhesive materials in 3T3 cells.

For 3T3 fibroblasts, the cytotoxicity order obtained of the filtered adhesive extracts was T1 (less cytotoxic) < Scotchbond Universal < Optibond Solo Plus (most cytotoxic). For MG-63 osteoblasts, the least toxic was also the T1 adhesive, while the most toxic was Scotchbond Universal. Despite the limitations of this in vitro study, we can conclude that the three adhesives present a dose-dependent effect. The filtration of the same extract, or its absence, has effects on the cell viability, as well as the alteration of cell type, with MG-63 being more sensitive in general. In this study, the T1 adhesive is the one with the greatest biocompatibility, and taking into account that it is still in the experimental stage, further studies should be carried out to evaluate other important aspects in clinical practice.

Author Contributions: I.B. and P.M. (Paulo Maurício); Methodology, S.B.; Software, P.M. (Paulo Mascarenhas); Validation, S.S.; I.B.; Writing—Review & Editing, I.B.; A.C.R.; P.M.: Funding Acquisition, I.B. All authors have read and agreed to the published version of the manuscript.

Funding: The graduate student's thesis program in Dental Medicine from the Cooperativa de Ensino Superior, CRL, Caparica, Portugal.

Informed Consent Statement: Not applicable.

Acknowledgments: This work was done for Sofia Santos's master degree in Dentistry and it was supported by Egas Moniz, Cooperativa de Ensino Superior CRL.

Conflicts of Interest: The authors declare no conflict of interest.

References

1. Massaro, H.; Zambelli, L.F.; Britto, A.A.D.; Vieira, R.P.; Ligeiro-de-Oliveira, A.P.; Andia, D.C.; Oliveira, M.T.; Lima, A.F. Solvent and hema increase adhesive toxicity and cytokine release from dental pulp cells. *Materials* **2019**, *12*, 2750. [CrossRef] [PubMed]
2. Goldberg, M. In vitro and in vivo studies on the toxicity of dental resin components: A review. *Clin. Oral Investig.* **2008**, *12*, 1–8. [CrossRef] [PubMed]

3. Tadin, A.; Gavić, L.; Galić, N. Biocompatibility of dental adhesives. In *Adhesives-Applications and Properties*; Materials Science; Rudawska, A., Ed.; IntechOpen: London, UK, 2016. [CrossRef]
4. Bandarra, S.; Mascarenhas, P.; Luís, A.R.; Catrau, M.; Bekman, E.; Ribeiro, A.C.; Félix, S.; Caldeira, J.; Barahona, I. In vitro and in silico evaluations of resin-based dental restorative material toxicity. *Clin. Oral Investig.* **2020**, *24*, 2691–2700. [CrossRef] [PubMed]

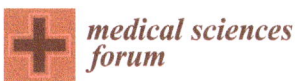

Proceeding Paper

Xerostomia and Medication in an Elderly Portuguese Population †

Inês Caetano Santos [1,2,3,*], **Fabrícia Martins** [1], **Kateryna Rudysh** [1], **Luís Proença** [1,2], **Ana Cristina Manso** [1,2], **Mário Polido** [1,2], **José João Mendes** [1,2] and **Helena Canhão** [3]

1. Instituto Universitário Egas Moniz, 2829-511 Caparica, Portugal; fabricia_ariana@gmail.com (F.M.); katerynarudysh@gmail.com (K.R.); luisfapro@gmail.com (L.P.); mansocristina@gmail.com (A.C.M.); mpolido@egasmoniz.edu.pt (M.P.); jmendes@egasmoniz.edu.pt (J.J.M.)
2. Centro de Investigação Interdisciplinar Egas Moniz (CiiEM), 2829-511 Caparica, Portugal
3. EpiDoc Unit, Chronic Diseases Research Centre (CEDOC), Nova Medical School, 1150-082 Lisboa, Portugal; helena.canhao@nms.unl.pt
* Correspondence: inescaetanosantos@gmail.com; Tel.: +351-91-657-5085
† Presented at the 5th International Congress of CiiEM—Reducing inequalities in Health and Society, Online, 16–18 June 2021.

Abstract: Xerostomia (dry mouth perception) is a condition that affects mastication, swallowing and speech and increases with age or can be the result of medication or some systemic diseases. The purpose of this exploratory study was to evaluate the prevalence of xerostomia in a local elderly population and its relationship with medication. It was verified that most of the participants have xerostomia, and from these, the majority take medication. Additionally, the prevalence of xerostomia varies with the type of medication taken. The presence of xerostomia was found to be significantly related to the number of medications taken.

Keywords: xerostomia; geriatrics; medication

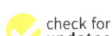

Citation: Santos, I.C.; Martins, F.; Rudysh, K.; Proença, L.; Manso, A.C.; Polido, M.; Mendes, J.J.; Canhão, H. Xerostomia and Medication in an Elderly Portuguese Population . *Med. Sci. Forum* **2021**, *5*, 8. https://doi.org/10.3390/msf2021005008

Academic Editors: Helena Barroso and Cidália Castro

Published: 12 July 2021

Publisher's Note: MDPI stays neutral with regard to jurisdictional claims in published maps and institutional affiliations.

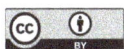

Copyright: © 2021 by the authors. Licensee MDPI, Basel, Switzerland. This article is an open access article distributed under the terms and conditions of the Creative Commons Attribution (CC BY) license (https://creativecommons.org/licenses/by/4.0/).

1. Introduction

The elderly population has been growing and is expected to continue to increase in the future [1]. Dry mouth perception (xerostomia) increases with age, affecting nearly 30% of the elderly, and it is most common in medicated patients or can be related to systemic diseases such as diabetes or Sjögren syndrome [2,3]. Studies identify many medications with xerogenic potential such as antidepressants, anticonvulsants, anticoagulants, antihypertensives, antihistamines or hypoglycemic medication [3,4]. The purpose of this study was to evaluate the prevalence of xerostomia in an elderly local population and determine the influence of medication on dry mouth perception.

2. Materials and Methods

This study, approved by a state-recognized ethical committee, included 80 elderly patients who attended a university dental clinic, in the Lisbon region urban area (Portugal), over a 3-month period. Inclusion criteria were: age 65+ years, being non-institutionalized and having signed an informed consent. Participants were distributed into four groups according to their age (years): 65–70, 71–75, 76–80 and 81+. Information was gathered through a questionnaire about xerostomia symptoms (yes/no) and medication taken. Medication was classified by pharmacological group (antihypertensives, antidiabetics, antidepressants, anticonvulsants, antihistamines, cytotoxic, anticoagulants and other medications), and the number of medications taken (1, 2 or 3+) was recorded. Data were analyzed through descriptive and inferential statistical methodologies. A significance level of 5% ($p = 0.05$) was considered.

3. Results and Discussion

3.1. Presence of Xerostomia in Each Age Group

From all the participants of this study, the majority (52.5%) have xerostomia symptoms. The age group 65–70 years revealed the highest prevalence of xerostomia (65.5%), followed by the 81+ years age group, with a xerostomia prevalence of 53.8%.

3.2. Presence of Xerostomia and Medication

From the participants with xerostomia symptoms, 90.5% take medication. In each pharmacological group, more than half of the medicated participants have xerostomia; however, a significant difference between different pharmacological groups was not identified ($p > 0.05$).

3.3. Presence of Xerostomia and Number of Medications Taken

The presence of xerostomia increased with the number of medications taken: 45.2% of the participants who have xerostomia take three or more medications, and only 9.5% who have xerostomia do not take any medication. The number of medications taken by participants with xerostomia was significantly higher when compared with patients without xerostomia ($p = 0.025$).

Several studies linked xerostomia with medication intake and showed that elderly patients that do not ingest any medication had a higher salivary flow rate than medicated patients [2]. Xerostomia-inducing medication interferes in the production of saliva or in the pathways responsible for salivary secretions, by direct or indirect action on the salivary glands [5,6]. An increase in medication leads to a reduction in salivary flow, affecting dry mouth perception, and the probability of having this symptom increases with additional medications, which demonstrates the synergistic effects of xerostomia-inducing medication in the elderly [2,5,6].

In conclusion, the majority of the participants in all age groups have xerostomia symptoms, and most of them take medication. Furthermore, these symptoms increased with the number of medications taken, which emphasizes the importance of oral preventive measures towards a better quality of life in the elderly.

Institutional Review Board Statement: The study was conducted according to the guidelines of the Declaration of Helsinki, and approved by the Ethics Committee of Instituto Universitário Egas Moniz (protocol code 896, approved on 30 July 2020).

Informed Consent Statement: Informed consent was obtained from all subjects involved in the study.

Data Availability Statement: The data presented in this study are available on request from the corresponding author. The data are not publicly available due to the research is still under development.

Conflicts of Interest: The authors declare no conflict of interest.

References

1. Van der Putten, G.J.; De Visschere, L.; Van der Maarel-Wierink, C.; Vanobbergen, J.; Schols, J. The importance of oral health in (frail) elderly people—A review. *Eur. Geriatr. Med.* **2013**, *4*, 339–344. [CrossRef]
2. Niklande, S.; Veas, L.; Fuentes, F.; Chiappini, G.; Barrera, C.; Marshal, M. Risk factors, hyposalivation and impact of xerostomia on oral health-related quality of life. *Braz. Oral Res.* **2017**, *31*, 1–9. [CrossRef]
3. Olofsson, H.; Ulander, E.L.; Gustafson, Y.; Hornsten, C. Association between socioeconomic and health factors and edentulism in people aged 65 and older—A population-based survey. *Scand. J. Public Health* **2017**, *46*, 690–698. [CrossRef] [PubMed]
4. Villa, A.; Nordio, F.; Gohel, A. A risk prediction model for xerostomia: A retrospective cohort study. *Gerodontology* **2016**, *33*, 562–568. [CrossRef] [PubMed]
5. Rogus-Pulia, N.M.; Gangnon, R.; Kind, A.; Connor, N.P.; Asthana, S. A Pilot Study of Perceived Mouth Dryness, Perceived Swallowing Effort, and Saliva Substitute Effects in Healthy Adults Across the Age Range. *Dysphagia* **2018**, *33*, 200–205. [CrossRef] [PubMed]
6. Shetty, S.R.; Bhowmick, S.; Castelino, R.; Babu, S. Drug induced xerostomia in elderly individuals: An institutional study. *Contemp. Clin. Dent.* **2012**, *3*, 173–175. [CrossRef] [PubMed]

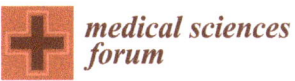

Proceeding Paper

Halitosis Self-Perception and Awareness among Periodontal Patients—An Exploratory Study †

Catarina Izidoro [1,2,*], **João Botelho** [2], **Vanessa Machado** [2], **Luis Proença** [3], **Ricardo Alves** [1,2] **and José João Mendes** [2]

1. Periodontology Department, Egas Moniz Dental Clinic, Egas Moniz—Cooperativa de Ensino Superior, 2829-511 Almada, Portugal; ralves@egasmoniz.edu.pt
2. Clinical Research Unit, Egas Moniz Interdisciplinary Research Center (CiiEM), Egas Moniz—Cooperativa de Ensino Superior, 2829-511 Almada, Portugal; jbotelho@egasmoniz.edu.pt (J.B.); vmachado@egasmoniz.edu.pt (V.M.); jmendes@egasmoniz.edu.pt (J.J.M.)
3. Quantitative Methods for Health Research Unit, CiiEM, Egas Moniz—Cooperativa de Ensino Superior, 2829-511 Almada, Portugal; lproenca@egasmoniz.edu.pt
* Correspondence: cizidoro@egasmoniz.edu.pt; Tel.: +351-91423-7448
† Presented at the 5th International Congress of CiiEM—Reducing Inequalities in Health and Society, Online, 16–18 June 2021.

Abstract: Halitosis is an unpleasant breath odor that interferes with self-confidence and with people's professional and social lives. The aim of this exploratory study was to evaluate the self-perception and awareness of oral malodor among patients with periodontitis.

Keywords: halitosis; self-perception; periodontitis; bad breath

1. Introduction

Halitosis or oral malodor is an unpleasant breath odor that interferes with one's quality of life [1,2]. As one of the main symptoms of periodontitis, halitosis often leads patients to seek treatment [3]. Several studies have addressed self-perceived halitosis among young people, but the number of studies on the self-perception of intra-oral halitosis in periodontitis patients is still scarce. The aim of this exploratory study was to assess the self-perception and awareness of oral malodor among periodontitis patients and to evaluate their relation to halitosis diagnosis.

2. Materials and Methods

This study was approved by the Egas Moniz Ethics Committee, in accordance with the Helsinki Declaration of 1975, as revised in 2013. Participants were consecutively recruited from the Periodontology Department at Egas Moniz Dental Clinic for periodontal assessment, between October 2019 and March 2021. The inclusion criteria were: periodontitis; 18 < age < 65, complying with the recommendations given for halitosis assessment and providing informed consent. Exclusion criteria were as follows: previous periodontal treatment; antibiotics within the last 4 weeks; history of radiotherapy or chemotherapy; extra-oral causes for halitosis; and pregnancy.

One calibrated examiner performed a full-mouth periodontal examination with a manual periodontal CP-12 probe (Hu-Friedy®, Chicago, IL, USA). Periodontitis was defined according to the AAP/EFP 2018 consensus [4]. Halitosis was diagnosed in two steps: (1) self-reported questionnaire, to exclude possible causes for extra-oral halitosis; self-perception of halitosis (using a visual analog scale of 10 cm); self-awareness was recorded as follows: (a) previously warned for bad breath; (b) whom might have informed them; and (c) self-perception for needing treatment for halitosis. Then, in step (2), volatile sulfur compounds (VSC) were quantified through a device (Halimeter®, Interscan Corp, Chatsworth, CA, USA), with less than 80 ppb denoted as no perceptible odor, and higher than 80 ppb denoted as halitosis [5]. Data were analyzed by descriptive and inferential methodologies. A significance level of 5% was established in the latter.

3. Results and Discussion

From a total of 117 participants, 57% females and 43% males, 84 were evaluated, regarding halitosis status, by VSC counting. From these, 46.4% were diagnosed as having halitosis (VSC > 80 ppb). Overall, self-perception for halitosis needing treatment (SPHNT) was low ($n = 42$, 51.2% from total) and awareness, brought to their attention by a third-party, was lower ($n = 32$, 38.1% from total). SPHNT was higher in the diagnosed halitosis group (57.9 vs. 45.5%) (Table 1); however, this difference was not found to be significant ($p = 0.261$). Simultaneously, the proportion of patients previously warned for their halitosis status (PWHS) was higher in that group (46.2 vs. 31.1%), albeit not significantly higher ($p = 0.157$). From these, the majority reported being alerted by a close family member (84.8%).

Table 1. Self-perception and awareness of halitosis as per the halitosis status through VSC count (SPHNT: self-perception for halitosis needing treatment; PWHS: previously warned for their halitosis tatus).

	No Halitosis (VSC ≤ 80 ppb)	Halitosis (VSC > 80 ppb)	p-Value
SPHNT ($n = 82$), (Yes /No), n (%)	20 (45.5)/24 (54.5)	22 (57.9)/16 (42.1)	0.261
PWHS ($n = 84$) (Yes/No), n (%)	14 (31.1)/31 (68.9)	18 (46.2)/21 (53.8)	0.157

A low rate of self-reported halitosis was found among these patients, and the majority were often informed by close family members. Most respondents indicated that they did not intend to seek treatment for bad breath. No association was found between self-perceived halitosis needing treatment or halitosis awareness and halitosis diagnosis.

Institutional Review Board Statement: The study was conducted according to the guidelines of the Declaration of Helsinki, and approved by Ethics Committee of EGAS MONIZ (n° 781, 26 June 2019).

Informed Consent Statement: Informed consent was obtained from all subjects involved in the study.

Acknowledgments: Acknowledgments addressed to the EMDC Periodontology Department, Egas Moniz—Cooperativa de Ensino Superior, CRL for all support.

Conflicts of Interest: The authors declare no conflict of interest.

References

1. Kukkamalla, D.; Cornelio, D.; Mahalinga Bhat, D.; Avadhani, D.; Goyal, D. HALITOSIS—A Social Malady. *IOSR-JDMS* **2014**, *13*, 55–61. [CrossRef]
2. Azodo, C.; Umoh, A. Self-perceived oral malodour among periodontal patients: Prevalence and associated factors. *Int. J. Med. Biomed. Res.* **2013**, *2*, 125–132. [CrossRef]
3. De Geest, S.; Laleman, I.; Teughels, W.; Dekeyser, C.; Quirynen, M. Periodontal Diseases as a Source of Halitosis: A Review of the Evidence and Treatment Approaches for Dentists and Dental Hygienists. *Periodontol. 2000* **2016**, *71*, 213–227. [CrossRef] [PubMed]
4. Tonetti, M.S.; Greenwell, H.; Kornman, K.S. Staging and Grading of Periodontitis: Framework and Proposal of a New Classification and Case Definition. *J. Periodontol.* **2018**, *45* (Suppl. 20), S149–S161. [CrossRef] [PubMed]
5. Donaldson, A.C.; Riggio, M.P.; Rolph, H.J.; Bagg, J.; Hodge, P.J. Clinical Examination of Subjects with Halitosis. *Oral Dis.* **2007**, *13*, 63–70. [CrossRef] [PubMed]

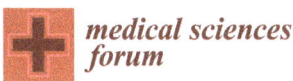

Proceeding Paper

Students, Medicines and Performance Consumption: The Online as a Source of Information and Sharing †

Catarina Egreja * and Noémia Lopes

Instituto Universitário Egas Moniz, 2829-511 Almada, Portugal; nlopes@egasmoniz.edu.pt
* Correspondence: cegreja@egasmoniz.edu.pt
† Presented at the 5th International Congress of CiiEM—Reducing Inequalities in Health and Society, Online, 16–18 June 2021.

Abstract: We aim to reflect on the online as a space to be taken into account in the analysis of sources of information about medicines, as a means of transmitting knowledge and practices among students, by presenting results of a content analysis based on material collected from blogs and internet forums. We conclude that sharing experiences is central to the validation of and willingness to use these resources. Considering the consequences that may arise from widespread use of the online as a source of information for therapeutic or performance purposes is important.

Keywords: medicines and supplements; online information sources; online sharing; performance enhancement in students

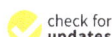

1. Introduction

Previous research concludes that the internet serves as a space for users to gain some expertise about medicines, being able to exchange ideas and ask questions. Users seek, in forums, to collect experiences from other users, and peer support in the search for a shared social identity; the higher the risk associated with health, the more the interest grows [1]. Online forums are valued because of the anonymity—being able to communicate without fear or worry and choosing how much information to share [2]. The growth of the internet and the increased use of forums means that users now have access to a wider range of views and opinions on their chosen topic [3,4].

The present exploratory approach reflects on the online as a space that should be taken into account in the analysis of sources of information on medicines, as a means of transmission of knowledge and practices among users, considering its potential and limits, by presenting the results of a content analysis based on material collected from blogs and internet forums. Objectively, the focus is on online information exchanges among high school and university students, on the consumption of medicines and natural products, with the purpose of improving the capacity to concentrate and memorize during exams. Although this is not a new research theme, its pertinence and topicality merit an opportunity to deepen the analysis.

2. Materials and Methods

The adopted methodology was qualitative content analysis. In order to find online information exchange practices on the consumption of medicines and natural products, the research process began by entering keywords into a search engine (Google). We did not intend to explore sites of pharmacies or companies linked to this area, nor to find sources of information that came from experts (doctors, pharmacists, etc.), but rather interactions between lay people, in this case, students. These were found in different forums and blogs, mostly of student associations, where participants sometimes asked questions about issues related to these consumptions.

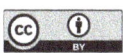

Next, we collected all the posts and respective comments of interest, which were categorized and examined relying on an analytic grid with the following structure, using the Maxqda software: (1) Sharing experiences-symptoms; therapeutic path (consumption, dosages, reactions...); request for help/clarification of doubts; (2) Sharing expert knowledge-diagnoses; recommended therapy; (3) Sharing lay knowledge-diagnoses; effects of medicines/supplements; consumption advices; advices of consultation with health professionals/others; other advices.

On the topic of consumption of performance-enhancing medicines and supplements among students, 93 conversation excerpts ranging from March 2015 to October 2020 were analysed.

3. Results and Discussion

The results show that one of the main reasons for students to use blogs and forums as a source of information is the possibility to share experiences (31.2%). One of the most frequent aspects concerns requests for help, mainly in order to obtain information and clarify doubts. Our analysis also indicates that students seek to know the opinion of their peers regarding the taking of supplements or medication to help them study, in order to obtain some kind of validation. This generates, in turn, a sharing of their own or other people's experiences, through the account of therapeutic paths (consumption, dosages, and reactions). However, the dimension of analysis with the highest proportion of content (63.4%) refers to the sharing of lay knowledge. In response to doubts or requests for information, the other participants in these virtual communities take the opportunity to offer their diagnoses, tell the effects of the medicines or supplements they think they know, or recommend ways of consumption. Finally, the dimension with the least expression is the sharing of expert knowledge (5.4%). Although this is not a common situation, some people copy information from package leaflets, a reliable site or scientific studies to present the effects and purposes of medicines in an expert way, not based on their personal convictions.

In conclusion, these means of access to information clearly reveal that the sharing of experiences is central to the validation and willingness to resort to such consumption. It is important to reflect on the consequences that may arise from the generalisation of these means as sources of information for therapeutic or performance purposes—not only in the case of students, but more broadly, by the population in general.

The study has limitations, such as the impossibility to know for sure if the online participants are, indeed, lay students, or the inability to characterize the sample. However, we believe that the aspects pointed out here justify a deepening of this line of research, also to strengthen current studies on the concept of medication literacy.

Institutional Review Board Statement: The study was conducted according to the guidelines of the Declaration of Helsinki, and approved by the Ethics Committee of Instituto Universitário Egas Moniz (protocol code CE 857/20.02.2020).

Informed Consent Statement: Not applicable.

Data Availability Statement: Not applicable.

Acknowledgments: This work is part of project ConPerLit (PTDC/SOC/30734/2017), funded by the Portuguese Foundation for Science and Technology.

Conflicts of Interest: The authors declare no conflict of interest.

References

1. Dresen, A.; Kläber, M.; Dietz, P. Use of performance-enhancing drugs and the Internet. Criminological reflections on a culture of communication in sport. *Sportwissenschaft* **2014**, *44*, 153–159. [CrossRef]
2. Fage-Butler, A.M.; Jensen, M.N. The Interpersonal Dimension of Online Patient Forums: How Patients Manage Informational and Relational Aspects in Response to Posted Questions. *Hermes J. Lang. Commun. Bus.* **2013**, *51*, 21–38. [CrossRef]

3. Tighe, B.; Dunn, M.; McKay, F.H.; Piatkowski, T. Information sought, information shared: Exploring performance and image enhancing drug user-facilitated harm reduction information in online forums. *Harm Reduct. J.* **2017**, *14*, 1–9. [CrossRef] [PubMed]
4. Rusu, I.A. Exchanging health advice in a virtual community: A story of tribalization. *J. Comp. Res. Anthropol. Sociol.* **2016**, *2*, 57–69.

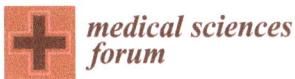

Proceeding Paper

Application of Cannabis Use Intention Questionnaire (CUIQ) to First Year University Students [†]

Inês Teodoro, Hugo Torres, Nuno Venâncio, Guilhermina Moutinho and Maria Deolinda Auxtero *

Centro de Investigação Interdisciplinar Egas Moniz (CiiEM), 2829-511 Almada, Portugal; inesgloria87@gmail.com (I.T.); hugofpgtorres@gmail.com (H.T.); nuno.venancio2000@gmail.com (N.V.); mgm.moutinho@gmail.com (G.M.)
* Correspondence: mauxtero@egasmoniz.edu.pt; Tel.: +351-212-946-823
† Presented at the 5th International Congress of CiiEM—Reducing inequalities in Health and Society, Online, 16–18 June 2021.

Abstract: Cannabis is the illegal drug most used worldwide. Its long-term use increases the risk of depression and schizophrenia, causing a major public health problem. A validated questionnaire was applied to first year students of Instituto Universitário Egas Moniz to assess their intention regarding cannabis use. They do not consider cannabis to be much associated with well-being, they slightly consider the opinion of relatives, and they show a low intent to use the drug, believing themselves to have strong self-control. Scores are above average for 18-y.o. Portuguese students, except for belief in self-control.

Keywords: Cannabis; CUIQ; university students; consumption; well-being; creativity

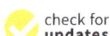

1. Introduction

Cannabis (CB) is the illegal drug most used and, in recent years, its consumption by adolescents and young adults has increased exponentially. In these groups, CB is mostly used recreationally, to achieve states of relaxation (61%) and feelings of joy (27%) [1]. In the long-term, CB increases the risk of depression, anxiety, and schizophrenia, representing an important public health issue [2]. A scale (cannabis use intention questionnaire—CUIQ) was designed and validated to measure attitudes towards CB consumption among young users (15–18 y.o.) in the EU, preferentially applied in the school environment [3]. The present study aimed to evaluate the intention of first year university students of Instituto Universitário Egas Moniz (IUEM) to consume CB, using the CUIQ.

2. Materials and Methods

The CUIQ is an anonymous questionnaire that was adapted for digital format through the Google Forms platform. It included four sections: (A) Attitude (At)—how consumption is judged to positively influence one's sense of well-being and creativity; (B) Subjective rule (SR)—the degree to which relatives would agree with consumption and valuation given to their opinion; (C) Self-efficacy (SE) towards abstinence and (D) Consumption intention (CI). All sections were assessed using a 5-point Likert scale, with 1 being the lowest degree of agreement or importance, and 5 the highest for sections A, B, and D. In section C, 1 corresponded to "not able at all" and 5 corresponded to "totally able". In May 2020, a cross-sectional study (approved by EM Ethics Committee) was conducted through the application of the questionnaire to 1st year, Portuguese students (who gave their electronic consent), of four courses of IUEM (Pharmacy-MICF, Forensic Sciences-LCFC, Dentistry-MIMD, and Nutrition-LCN). Data were processed with Microsoft Excel Software version 16.48 using the template supplied in the 'Application and correction manual for the CUIQ' for Portugal [3]. Mean scores for the IUEM and for each course were compared with the scale created for Portugal (18 years) for each section.

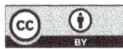

3. Results and Discussion

Of the 122 respondents, aged 18 to 22 years, 45.9% (*n* = 56) were 18 years old students. Since the questionnaire applied is validated for people aged between 15 and 18 years, all participants aged over 18 were excluded. Hence, the validated sample included 8 MICF students, 8 LCN students, 17 from MIMD, and 23 LCFC students. The average results obtained are presented in Figure 1a,b.

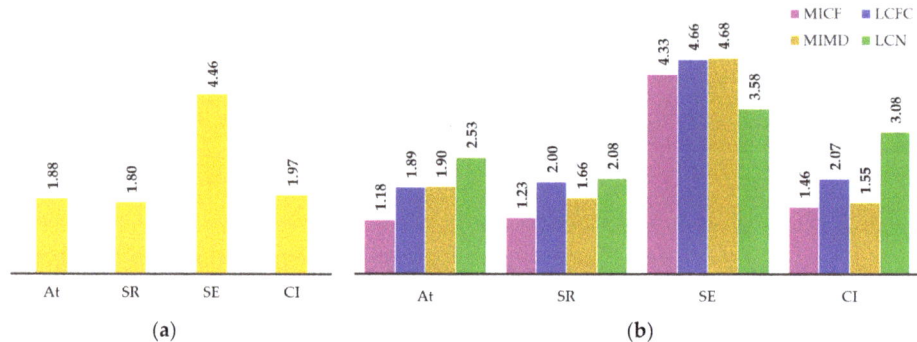

Figure 1. (**a**) Average score of the global sample (*n* = 56); (**b**) Average score by course. At (Attitude); SR (Subjective rule); SE (Self-efficacy); CI (Consumption intention).

The average score in At was 1.88 points which is positioned between percentile 50 and 60. Hence, our sample is slightly above the average group of 18 years-old in terms of score for positive At towards CB consumption. The mean score for section B was 1.80 points, falling within the 30% of individuals who have a higher score towards SR. The average score in SE was 4.46 points, positioning our sample within the 60% of young people of their age that have less difficulty in maintaining the attitude of abstinence. Finally, the average score in section D was 1.97 points, corresponding to a percentile between 60 and 70, which means that it is included within the 40% that have a higher score, indicating higher CI. Figure 1b illustrates the mean score of each course group. LCN students scored the highest values for At, SR, and CI. This suggests that they believe that CB consumption positively influences their well-being, and show higher intention to consume it, as well as more difficulty in maintaining abstinence. On the other hand, it is easier for LCFC and MIMD students to keep longer abstinence periods. MICF students have lower intention to consume than the others, although they take less into consideration relatives' opinion about the consumption of CB.

Our sample is above the national average for all scores but SE. Students revealed a high perception of the SE to abstain, and lower intention to consume CB which is in agreement with the low positive attitude towards CB consumption. The opinion of relatives is not overvalued.

Institutional Review Board Statement: The study was conducted according to the guidelines of the Declaration of Helsinki, and approved by the Ethics Committee of Egas Moniz (protocol code 879, 27 May 2021).

Informed Consent Statement: Informed consent was obtained from all subjects involved in the study.

Data Availability Statement: The data presented in this study are available on request from the corresponding author. The data are not publicly available due to privacy restrictions.

Acknowledgments: We would like to thank all the participants and our colleagues for sharing their results.

Conflicts of Interest: The authors declare that there are no conflict of interest.

References

1. Herruzo, C.; Pino, M.J.; Lucena, V.; Herruzo, J. Perceptual Styles and Cannabis Consumption Prediction in Young People. *Int. J. Environ. Res. Public Health* **2020**, *17*, 288. [CrossRef] [PubMed]
2. United Nations Office on Drugs and Crime. *World Drug Report 2019*; United Nations Publication: New York, NY, USA, 2019; pp. 1–76.
3. European Commission CAPPYC (Cannabis Abuse Prevention Program for Young Consumers). Available online: http://cappyc.eu (accessed on 16 May 2020).

Proceeding Paper

Intimate Partner Violence Risk Assessment in Victims Information and Assistance Office [†]

Iris Almeida [1,2,3,4,*], Ana Rita Pires [1], Carolina Nobre [4], Joana Marques [4] and Patrícia Oliveira [1]

1. Instituto Universitário Egas Moniz (IUEM), Egas Moniz-Cooperativa de Ensino Superior, Crl., 2829-511 Almada, Portugal; anaritaf_pires@hotmail.com (A.R.P.); patriciasofia_27@hotmail.com (P.O.)
2. Laboratório de Psicologia (LabPSI), Centro de Investigação Interdisciplinar Egas Moniz (CiiEM), 2829-511 Almada, Portugal
3. Laboratório de Ciências Forenses e Psicológicas Egas Moniz (LCFPEM), 2829-511 Almada, Portugal
4. Gabinete de Informação e Atendimento à Vítima, 1990-097 Lisboa, Portugal; carolinanobrepsic@gmail.com (C.N.); joanaromba@hotmail.com (J.M.)
* Correspondence: ialmeida@egasmoniz.edu.pt
† Presented at the 5th International Congress of CiiEM—Reducing inequalities in Health and Society, Online, 16–18 June 2021.

Abstract: The purpose of this paper is to demonstrate the work developed by the Victims Information and Assistance Office (GIAV), and its role as technical advisor to the Lisbon Public Prosecutor's Office, specifically about Intimate Partner Violence (IPV) risk assessment. GIAV plays a key role in assisting the Public Prosecutor's Office as the main response to cases with higher complexity and it provides support about measures to protect victims. The sample (n = 258) is derived from the IPV risk assessments of GIAV. Results show us that moderate and higher risk are the most common levels in IPV risk assessment and main risk factors. Defendants had more beliefs about IPV than victims.

Keywords: Intimate Partner Violence; risk assessment; public prosecutor's office

1. Introduction

Forensic psychological assessment, specifically violence risk assessment, is an essential element in the practice of forensic psychology [1] and plays a crucial role in criminal justice system, helping it to make decisions [2]. IPV risk assessment is an essential element in offender's evaluation. Consequently, it is possible to apply the most appropriate intervention to prevent violence, protecting victims, and re-socializing offenders [3]. This assessment identifies risk factors such as criminal history, social and situational factors, and psychological variables [3]. IPV risk assessment includes semi-structured interviews and forensic psychological assessment tools which allows the identification of risk factors [4].

2. Materials and Methods

The sample (n = 258) is derived from the IPV risk assessments of GIAV (2011–2020). We evaluate 115 victims: 107 women and 8 men, aged between 17 and 73 years old (M = 44.68, sd = 12.50); 106 defendants: 100 men and 6 women, aged between 17 and 81 years old (M = 46.33, sd = 12.74); and 36 victims and defendants simultaneously: 19 men and 17 women, aged between 23 and 58 years old (M = 41.75, sd = 10.47). The relationship between victims and defendants are: 85 married; 61 ex-boyfriend/girlfriend; 36 ex-spouses; 31 ex-partners; 31 partners; 10 boyfriend/girlfriend; 2 lovers. Data was collected from lawsuits, semi-structured interviews, collateral information, and clinical and forensic assessment tools (e.g., SARA; ECVC; AQ).

3. Results and Discussion

In the risk assessments, most of the cases presented a moderate risk (39.5%), followed by high risk (21.7%) and low risk (17.4%). IPV risk factors are associated with extreme minimization or denial of spousal assault history (72.5%); recent relationship problems (71.4%); former physical assault (64.8%); severe and/or sexual assault (54.7%); past sexual assault/sexual jealousy (50%); personality disorder with anger, impulsivity or behavioural instability (47.7%); attitudes that support or condone spousal assault (47.7%); recent escalation in frequency or severity of assault (46.1%). Defendants had more beliefs about IPV than victims, especially in: Legitimization and trivialization of minor violence (e.g., insulting, slapping) ($M = 28.02$; $sd = 11.30$), legitimization of violence by the preservation of family privacy (e.g., what goes on between a couple only concerns the couple) ($M = 14.03$; $sd = 5.79$) and global beliefs ($M = 77.09$; $sd = 29.02$). Table 1 shows the correlations between individuals' legitimization beliefs (ECVC) and aggression (AQ). The results show us that legitimizing beliefs are associated with IPV.

Table 1. Correlations between legitimizing beliefs of violence and type of aggression.

	Legitimization of Minor Violence	Legitimization by Women's Conduct	Legitimization by External Causes	Legitimization by the Preservation of Family Privacy	Total BELIEFS
Psysical agression	0.248 **	0.214 *	0.281 **	0.185 *	0.250 **
Anger	0.261 **	0.218 *	0.256 **	0.187 *	0.251 **
Hostility	0.412 **	0.370 **	0.383 **	0.453 **	0.430 **
Total AQ score	0.405 **	0.346 **	0.383 **	0.349 **	0.400 **

** $p < 0.01$; * $p < 0.05$.

The work developed by GIAV allows the understanding of IPV risk assessment, through the articulation between Forensic Psychology and Law for a more informed decision making. The main goal of IPV risk assessment is the prevention and development of management strategies to minimize risk and try to identify factors that may contribute to the violent behavior supporting the criminal justice system in allocating more appropriate measures (e.g., sentence, intervention).

Institutional Review Board Statement: This study is part of a protocol established among the Portuguese Public Prosecutor's Office and Egas Moniz—Higher Education School to assess and analyze the characteristics of victims and offenders in the field of Violence. The strictness of ethical and deontological principles is safeguarded once criminal records have been restricted access by law (including judicial secrecy). Therefore, all assessed subjects gave their informed consent, and their data were processed anonymously.

Informed Consent Statement: All ethical issues were considered due to the sensitive nature of the detailed data, the respective informed consent, confidentiality limits, and information about the ethics and technician's impartiality.

Data Availability Statement: Data sharing not applicable because part of information derives from criminal records.

Conflicts of Interest: The authors declare no conflict of interest.

References

1. Simões, M.R. Potencialidades e limites do uso de instrumentos no processo de avaliação psicológica. *Psicol. Educ. Cult.* **2005**, *9*, 237–264.
2. Laboratório de Ciências Forenses e Psicológicas Egas Moniz–Gabinete de Psicologia Forense. *Manual Para Agentes Qualificados/As de Atendimento à Vítima*. Available online: https://www.egasmoniz.com.pt/media/119234/Maria-Manual.pdf (accessed on 29 April 2021).
3. Almeida, I.; Soeiro, C. Avaliação de risco de violência conjugal: Versão para polícias (SARA: PV). *Anál. Psicol.* **2010**, *1*, 179–192. [CrossRef]
4. Gonçalves, R.A.; Cunha, O.; Dias, A.R.C. Avaliação Psicológica de Agressores Conjugais. In *Manual de Psicologia Forense: Contextos, Práticas e Desafios*; Matos, M., Gonçalves, R.A., Machado, C., Eds.; Psiquilíbrios: Braga, Portugal, 2011; pp. 70–71.

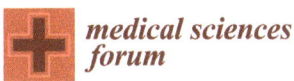

Proceeding Paper

The Forensic Psychology Role: Technical Advisor Office [†]

Iris Almeida [1,2,3,*], Ana Ramalho [3], Joana Costa [3] and Ricardo Ventura Baúto [1,2,3]

1 Instituto Universitário Egas Moniz (IUEM), Egas Moniz-Cooperativa de Ensino Superior, Crl., 2829-511 Almada, Portugal; rbauto.lcfpem@egasmoniz.edu.pt
2 Laboratório de Psicologia (LabPSI), Centro de Investigação Interdisciplinar Egas Moniz (CiiEM), 2829-511 Almada, Portugal
3 Laboratório de Ciências Forenses e Psicológicas Egas Moniz (LCFPEM), 2829-511 Almada, Portugal; acnramalho@gmail.com (A.R.); jcosta.lcfpem@egasmoniz.edu.pt (J.C.)
* Correspondence: ialmeida@egasmoniz.edu.pt
† Presented at the 5th International Congress of CiiEM—Reducing inequalities in Health and Society, Online, 16–18 June 2021.

Abstract: The purpose of this paper is to demonstrate the work developed by Technical Advisor Office (GAT) and its role as technical advisor to the West Lisbon Public Prosecutor's Office. GAT was established in partnership with Egas Moniz Higher Education School and West Lisbon Public Prosecutor's Office. GAT plays a crucial role in assisting the Public Prosecutor's Office as the main response to cases with higher complexity, and it provides support about measures to protect victims. GAT integrates the forensic psychologist narrowly and directly in monitoring processes in the judicial system, allowing a greater understanding of the phenomenon and facilitating decision-making by the Public Prosecutor's Office.

Keywords: forensic psychology; technical advisor; public prosecutor's office

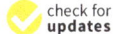

Citation: Almeida, I.; Ramalho, A.; Costa, J.; Baúto, R.V. The Forensic Psychology Role: Technical Advisor Office. *Med. Sci. Forum* **2021**, *5*, 13. https://doi.org/10.3390/msf2021005013

Academic Editors: Helena Barroso and Cidália Castro

Published: 20 July 2021

Publisher's Note: MDPI stays neutral with regard to jurisdictional claims in published maps and institutional affiliations.

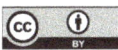

Copyright: © 2021 by the authors. Licensee MDPI, Basel, Switzerland. This article is an open access article distributed under the terms and conditions of the Creative Commons Attribution (CC BY) license (https://creativecommons.org/licenses/by/4.0/).

1. Introduction

The relevance of psychology in the Portuguese Justice System has been gaining projection in recent decades, emerging from the articulation between the two areas of knowledge, Forensic Psychology as a scientific discipline and with scope to allow its specialization [1,2]. Considering that the object of Forensic Psychology is the evaluation of human behaviour associated with the different contexts of justice's action and except for the importance that it has been acquiring at the level of the investigation phase, the presence of the psychologist in the justice system is configured as a technical element, capable of assisting in the intervention processes associated with victims, offenders, magistrates or other judicial officials. The evolution of criminal and procedural legislation has highlighted the role of psychological sciences as an asset in different areas of judicial decision. To note that the role of Forensic Psychology has been the most pertinence in the investigation phases as a tool to aid judicial decision, verifying through statistical analyses promoted in several studies [3]. That expert reports drawn up by forensic psychologists are mostly welcomed by the magistrates [1]. More recently, with legislative and regulatory reforms, new competencies and dynamics of intervention and prevention of forensic psychologists have emerged. In this sense, the forensic psychologist appears in this institution with the function of fulfilling the needs evoked by the justice system itself, seeking under its specific competencies to respond to the needs evidenced in this context. Thus, the Technical Advisor Office gives an integrated and direct response by inserting the forensic psychologist in the justice system, allowing a faster speed in the decision-making processes that result from the action of the Public Prosecutor's Office.

2. Materials and Methods

In 2019 and 2020, GAT had intervention in 231 criminal cases in West Lisbon Public Prosecutor's Office. Data was collected from lawsuits, semi-structured interviews of the victims and defendants, collateral information, and clinical and forensic assessment tools. All ethical issues have been taken due to the sensitive nature of the detailed data and the respective informed consentient, the confidentiality limits, and information about the ethics and technician's impartiality.

3. Results and Discussion

In 2019, it was possible to verify that 96 interventions were carried out with victims of crime (74 women and 22 men). In 2020, it was possible to verify that 201 interventions were carried out with victims of crime (128 women and 73 men). Article 271 of the Portuguese Code of Criminal Procedure allows the prosecutors and the inquiring judge to record the victim's testimony and use it during the future trial. This procedure, called future memory statements, prevents the victim from being exposed months or years later to the memories of a traumatic event. To minimize this, it is necessary to inform and prepare the victims for this diligence, explaining the court procedures. In 2019, to follow-ups in procedural acts, it was found that 33 occurred in future memory statements, and 26 other acts (e.g., monitoring of victims in recognition of suspects; making statements by prosecutors). In forensic psychological assessment: 19 psychological assessments; 7 forensic psychological assessment (with subsequent follow-up in future memory statements); 6 domestic violence risk assessments; 5 domestic violence risk assessments (with subsequent follow-up in future memory statements). In 2020, 86 psychological assessments; 16 forensic psychological evaluations with subsequent follow-up in procedural acts (future memory statements, inquiry, trial hearing and parent conferences); and two violence risk assessments. Follow-up in procedural acts found that 28 due diligence took place (e.g., making statements by prosecutors) and 26 future memory statements. GAT seeks to be an asset in straightforward advice to the justice system, having its main premise, the action close to the victim, with active support in judicial decision making. The demand for services provided in the superior support of victims of crime is the fundamental basis of GAT.

Institutional Review Board Statement: This study is part of a protocol established among the Portuguese Public Prosecutor's Office and Egas Moniz—Higher Education School to assess and analyze the characteristics of victims and offenders in the field of Violence. The strictness of ethical and deontological principles is safeguarded once criminal records have been restricted access by law (including judicial secrecy). Therefore, all assessed subjects gave their informed consent, and their data were processed anonymously.

Informed Consent Statement: All ethical issues were considered due to the sensitive nature of the detailed data, the respective informed consent, confidentiality limits, and information about the ethics and technician's impartiality.

Data Availability Statement: Data sharing not applicable because part of information derives from criminal records.

Conflicts of Interest: The authors declare no conflict of interest.

References

1. Gonçalves, R.A. Psicologia forense em Portugal: Uma história de responsabilidades e desafios. *Anál. Psicol.* **2010**, *28*, 107–115. [CrossRef]
2. Matos, M.; Gonçalves, R.A.; Machado, C. *Manual de Psicologia Forense: Contextos, Práticas e Desafios*; Coords: Psiquilíbrios, Portugal, 2011.
3. Castro, A.J.; Martins, A.S.; Machado, C.; Gonçalves, R.A. *Perícias Psicológicas, Sentenças Judiciais: Que Relação? Poster Apresentado no Congresso Internacional de Psicologia Forense*; Universidade do Minho: Braga, Portugal, 2006.

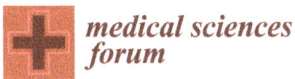

Proceeding Paper

Candida spp. Colonization among Intensive Care Unit Patients, Preliminary Results †

Teresa Nascimento [1,2,*], João Inácio [2,3], Isabel Ferreira [4], Priscila Diaz [4], Paulo Freitas [4] and Helena Barroso [1]

1. Centro de investigação interdisciplinar Egas Moniz (CiiEM), Instituto Universitário Egas Moniz, 2829-511 Almada, Portugal; mhbarroso@egasmoniz.edu.pt
2. Unidade de Microbiologia Médica, Global Health and Tropical Medicine (GHTM), Instituto de Higiene e Medicina Tropical Universidade Nova de Lisboa, 1349-008 Lisboa, Portugal; j.inacio@ihmt.unl.pt
3. School of Pharmacy and Biomolecular Sciences, University of Brighton, Brighton BN2 4GJ, UK
4. Hospital Prof. Doutor Fernando da Fonseca, 2720-276 Amadora, Portugal; isabel.p.ferreira@hff.min-saude.pt (I.F.); priscila.diaz@hff.min-saude.pt (P.D.); paulo.freitas@hff.min-saude.pt (P.F.)

* Correspondence: tnascimento@egasmoniz.edu.pt; Tel.: +351-212946744
† Presented at the 5th International Congress of CiiEM—Reducing inequalities in Health and Society, Online, 16–18 June 2021.

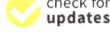

Abstract: *Candida* spp. colonization is recognized as a major risk factor for invasive candidiasis. To assess patient colonization, upon admission and during their stay in intensive care units (ICU), a surveillance study has been conducted since January 2020, in the Lisbon area of Portugal. A total of 219 swab samples were obtained from 113 ICU patients. The yeast identification was conducted by microbiological conventional and molecular methods. Upon admission to the ICU, 27% of patients were already colonized, and 17% became colonized during their ICU stay. *Candida albicans* was the most isolated species. These results may offer an opportunity for prevention of candidemia.

Keywords: yeasts; surveillance; colonization; identification; *Candida* spp.

Citation: Nascimento, T.; Inácio, J.; Ferreira, I.; Diaz, P.; Freitas, P.; Barroso, H. *Candida* spp. Colonization among Intensive Care Unit Patients, Preliminary Results. *Med. Sci. Forum* **2021**, *5*, 14. https://doi.org/10.3390/msf2021005014

Academic Editors: Helena Barroso and Cidália Castro

Published: 20 July 2021

Publisher's Note: MDPI stays neutral with regard to jurisdictional claims in published maps and institutional affiliations.

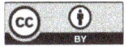

Copyright: © 2021 by the authors. Licensee MDPI, Basel, Switzerland. This article is an open access article distributed under the terms and conditions of the Creative Commons Attribution (CC BY) license (https://creativecommons.org/licenses/by/4.0/).

1. Introduction

Candida is the most common genus of commensal fungi present in different mycobiomes [1]. These yeasts are commensal in healthy humans and can cause systemic infection in situations where the host is immunocompromised. Of these, previous *Candida* spp. colonization stands out as the main predisposing factor for infection [2]. Colonized patients may also constitute reservoirs of species that are multidrug-resistant to antifungal drugs and that enhance horizontal transmission [2]. The literature on mycological epidemiological data in the intensive care unit (ICU) setting in Portugal is scarce. The aim of this work is to assess patients with *Candida* spp. colonization in an ICU environment.

2. Materials and Methods

To examine the presence of *Candida* spp., an ongoing surveillance study has been conducted since January 2020 in the ICUs of a tertiary hospital, Prof. Doutor Fernando Fonseca Hospital (HFF), in the Lisbon area of Portugal. The research has been conducted upon the admission of patients to the ICU and continues for the duration of stay (5 and 8 days). As a measure of the hospital control infection practice, chlorhexidine baths were taken during the swab collection time. Inclusion criteria include at least three risk factors for *Candida* spp. colonization/infection. All patients under the age of 18, pregnant women, and mentally disabled individuals were not included in the study. The sampling of each patient was performed by a non-invasive procedure using an axillary/inguinal combine swab. Identification of isolates was determined at a species level based on microbiological conventional and molecular methods.

3. Results and Discussion

A total of 219 composite axilla and inguinal swabs were obtained from 113 ICU patients. A total of 113 samples were collected on admission day, and 106 were collected during the time that the patients were in the ICU: 76 on 5th day and 30 on 8th day of ICU stay.

Of the 219 samples collected, 71 (32%) yielded *Candida* species. The most commonly recovered species were the *Candida albicans* (49%), *Candida parapsilosis* (34%), and *Candida glabrata* complexes (8%). No emerging rare species, such as *Candida auris*, were detected. Upon admission to the ICU, 27% (31/113) of the patients were already colonized with yeasts, and 17% (18/106) became colonized after admission. During their ICU stay, 38% (40/106) of patients were colonized, even after two chlorhexidine baths. Persistent colonization occurred in 27% (8/30) of patients who had three collections performed; in 50% of them, colonization persisted with *C. albicans*. High colonization (>10^3 CFU/mL) was shown in 18% of patients (20/113) at ICU admission. A colonization reduction was observed in only in 7% (2/30) of patients with an 8-day stay in the ICU.

Results from samples yielding *Candida* were consistent with the observations of other investigators, but we found lower rates upon admission [3]. Available studies in Portugal have focused on *Candida* spp. isolates in blood cultures [4,5]. The investigators also showed a prevalence of *C. albicans* but evidenced a change in the distribution of the isolated *Candida* species, with an increase in the proportion of *C. glabrata* [4]. This was not observed in our preliminary results. This study is the first attempt to systematically characterize the extent of *Candida* spp. colonization in ICU patients in Portugal. It may be necessary to conduct a nationally representative study of *Candida* spp. prevalence in the ICU, which can be guided by experience from this pilot.

Institutional Review Board Statement: Approved by Institutional Ethical Board of the Prof. Doutor Fernando Fonseca Hospital on 13/11/2019 (54/2019).

Informed Consent Statement: Informed consent was obtained from all subjects involved in the study.

Acknowledgments: The authors thank funding by CiiEM, Egas Moniz, Cooperativa de Ensino Superior, CRL.

Conflicts of Interest: The authors declare no conflict of interest.

References

1. Tiew, P.Y.; Mac Aogain, M.; Ali, N.A.B.M.; Thng, K.X.; Goh, K.; Lau, K.J.X.; Chotirmall, S.H. The mycobiome in health and disease: Emerging concepts, methodologies and challenges. *Mycopathologia* **2020**, *185*, 207–231. [CrossRef]
2. Keighley, C.L.; Pope, A.; Marriott, D.J.E.; Chapman, B.; Bak, N.; Daveson, K.; Hajkowicz, K.; Halliday, C.; Kennedy, K.; Kidd, S.; et al. Risk factors for candidaemia: A prospective multi-centre case-control study. *Mycoses* **2021**, *64*, 257–263. [CrossRef] [PubMed]
3. Ahmad, S.; Khan, Z.; Mustafa, A.S.; Khan, Z.U. Epidemiology of *Candida* colonization in an intensive care unit of a teaching hospital in Kuwait. *Med. Mycol.* **2003**, *41*, 487–493. [CrossRef] [PubMed]
4. Pinto-Magalhães, S.; Martins, A.; Lacerda, S.; Filipe, R.; Prista-Leão, B.; Pinheiro, D.; Silva-Pinto, A.; Santos, L. Candidemia in a Portuguese tertiary care hospital: Analysis of a 2-year period. *J. Mycol. Med.* **2019**, *29*, 320–324. [CrossRef] [PubMed]
5. Faria-Ramos, I.; Neves-Maia, J.; Ricardo, E.; Santos-Antunes, J.; Silva, A.T.; Costa-de-Oliveira, S.; Cantón, E.; Rodrigues, A.G.; Pina-Vaz, C. Species distribution and in vitro antifungal susceptibility profiles of yeast isolates from invasive infections during a Portuguese multicenter survey. *Eur. J. Clin. Microbiol. Infect. Dis.* **2014**, *33*, 2241–2247. [CrossRef] [PubMed]

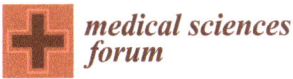

Proceeding Paper

Influence of the Infill Geometry of 3D-Printed Tablets on Drug Dissolution †

Nuno Venâncio [1], Gabriela G. Pereira [2], João F. Pinto [2] and Ana I. Fernandes [1,*]

1. CiiEM, Interdisciplinary Research Center Egas Moniz, Instituto Universitário Egas Moniz, 2829-511 Almada, Portugal; nuno.venancio2000@gmail.com
2. iMed.ULisboa–Research Institute for Medicines, Faculdade de Farmácia, Universidade de Lisboa, 1649-003 Lisboa, Portugal; garrastazugp@farm-id.pt (G.G.P.); jfpinto@ff.ul.pt (J.F.P.)
* Correspondence: aifernandes@egasmoniz.edu.pt; Tel.: +351-212946823
† Presented at the 5th International Congress of CiiEM—Reducing Inequalities in Health and Society, Online, 16–18 June 2021.

Abstract: Patient-centric therapy is especially important in pediatrics and may be attained by three-dimensional printing. Filaments containing 30% w/w of theophylline were produced by hot-melt extrusion and printed using fused deposition modelling to produce tablets. Here, preliminary results evaluating the effect of infill geometry (cross, star, grid) on drug content and release are reported.

Keywords: 3D-printing; theophylline; tablets; infill geometry; dissolution

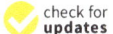

Citation: Venâncio, N.; Pereira, G.G.; Pinto, J.F.; Fernandes, A.I. Influence of the Infill Geometry of 3D-Printed Tablets on Drug Dissolution. *Med. Sci. Forum* **2021**, *5*, 15. https://doi.org/10.3390/msf2021005015

Academic Editors: Helena Barroso and Cidália Castro

Published: 20 July 2021

Publisher's Note: MDPI stays neutral with regard to jurisdictional claims in published maps and institutional affiliations.

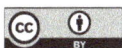

Copyright: © 2021 by the authors. Licensee MDPI, Basel, Switzerland. This article is an open access article distributed under the terms and conditions of the Creative Commons Attribution (CC BY) license (https://creativecommons.org/licenses/by/4.0/).

1. Introduction

Additive manufacturing, also known as 3D-printing (3DP), is gaining relevance in the manufacturing of personalized medicines, mainly of tablets (TAB), using fused deposition modelling (FDM). This technique requires prior drug incorporation in the matrix (e.g., thermoplastic polymers) and the production of filaments (FIL) through hot-melt extrusion (HME). FIL are in turn fed into the 3D-printer, molten and deposited layer-by-layer to build the dosage form [1]. The extrudability and printability of FIL depend on the raw materials (adjusted qualitatively and quantitatively, as required) and the processing conditions [1]. Since both HME and FDM rely on the fusion of the matrix, the heat stability of the drug is paramount.

The customization of medicines in pediatrics is critical, as one needs to repeatedly adjust the dose according to age, body weight or surface area as the child grows and to achieve well-defined drug release kinetics. This work evaluates how the infill geometry of 3D-printed TAB impacts drug content and release.

2. Materials and Methods

Theophylline (TEO; Sigma Aldrich) was chosen as a model drug (m.p. 270–274 °C). The thermoplastic matrix comprised hydroxypropylcellulose (HPC; m.p. 371 °C; Ashland), Soluplus® (SLP; BASF), and magnesium stearate (MgS; Roic Farma).

Drug-loaded FIL (30:54:15:1 % w/w–TEO:HPC:SLP:MgS) were obtained by HME, (ϕ1.5 mm nozzle; temperature 130 ± 5 °C) using a single-screw extruder (Noztek Touch, Noztek); drug-free FIL were used as controls. TAB were printed (extrusion temperature: 220 °C; extrusion speed: 90 mm/s; travelling speed: 150 mm/s; number of shells: 2; infill geometry: cross, star, and grid (without top and bottom); layer thickness: 0.20 mm) with a FDM 3D printer (Delta WASP 20 40 Turbo 2, Wasp); TAB dimensions and infill were designed with 3D Sprint Software (3D Systems).

Physical mixtures of materials, FIL and TAB were characterized by infrared (FTIR; Bruker), differential scanning calorimetry (DSC; TA Instruments), and X-ray diffractometry (XRPD; X'Pert PRO PANalytical). Dissolution of the TAB was evaluated for up to 24 h, using the paddle method (n = 3; 50 rpm, 900 mL HCl; 37 ± 0.5°C; Erweka DT600). TEO was quantified by HPLC (λ = 272 nm; HP 1100) [2].

3. Results and Discussion

Initial experiments have shown that the qualitative and quantitative composition of the chosen polymeric matrix possesses adequate plasticity and lubrication, enabling successful HME and FDM 3DP.

The uniformity of drug distribution in the FIL (samples from ends and middle of the extrudate) was ascertained as 98.15 ± 3.35% of the theoretical amount of TEO, also confirming drug stability during HME. Moreover, the heating of TEO at the printing temperature did not reveal degradation peaks in HPLC. TEO suffered partial amorphization caused by HME, a phenomenon strengthened during the FDM printing of the TAB, as ascertained by disappearance of the drug peaks in DSC and XRPD.

To evaluate the impact of geometry on dissolution, TAB of different infill geometry (cross, star, and grid, without a top and bottom; Figure 1) were 3D-printed and characterized (Table 1).

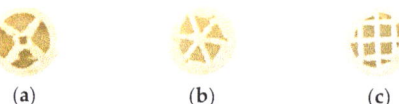

(a)   (b)   (c)

Figure 1. Infill geometry of the 3D-printed TAB: (**a**) cross; (**b**) star; (**c**) grid.

Table 1. Features of 3D-printed TAB [1].

TAB Infill Geometry	Diameter (mm)	Height (mm)	Mass (mg)	Drug Content [2] (mg)	Drug Recovery [3] (%)
Cross	12.00 ± 0.50	3.03 ± 0.02	196.80 ± 4.32	19.83 ± 1.74	33.54 ± 1.92
Star	12.50 ± 0.50	3.01 ± 0.01	246.10 ± 6.30	28.23 ± 1.07	37.72 ± 0.31
Grid	12.25 ± 0.73	3.03 ± 0.01	243.20 ± 9.14	27.44 ± 0.27	37.52 ± 0.42

[1] Results are mean ± standard deviation; n = 10 for diameter, height, and mass; n = 3 for content. [2] Amount of TEO quantified per tablet. [3] Expressed as percentage of the theoretical amount of TEO considering the TAB mass.

TAB dimensions, mass, and drug content were uniform. The star and grid TAB were equivalent; the cross showed significantly lower mass. Drug content was consistently below the theoretical value, but no degradation or interaction of TEO with the matrix was found by FTIR. Spontaneous micellization of the polymeric matrix (e.g., SOL) may account for the unavailability of the drug for quantitation.

In vitro drug release did not reveal significant differences related to infill geometry between the star and grid shapes since the surface area of exposure to the dissolution media did not seem to have a sufficient enough difference to impact the dissolution profile. For the cross geometry, the larger void spaces account for the higher accessibility of water to the structure, as well as slightly faster and more complete drug dissolution ($\approx$100% at 3 h); the star and grid show higher mass and thicker walls, so the matrix effect on slowing drug release is more marked ($\approx$95% after 4–5 h).

Further in-depth studies are warranted to fully understand and characterize the systems and to explore the impact of geometry on dissolution.

Acknowledgments: This work was supported by Fundação para a Ciência e a Tecnologia [grant number PTDC/CTM-CTM/30949/2017 (Lisboa 010145 Feder 030949)].

Conflicts of Interest: The authors declare no conflict of interest.

References

1. Pereira, G.C.; Figueiredo, S.; Fernandes, A.I.; Pinto, J.F. Polymer selection for hot-melt extrusion coupled to fused deposition modelling in pharmaceutics. *Pharmaceutics* **2020**, *12*, 795. [CrossRef] [PubMed]
2. Okwuosa, T.C.; Pereira, B.C.; Arafat, B.; Cieszynska, M.; Isreb, A.; Alhnan, M.A. Fabricating a shell-core delayed release tablet using dual FDM 3D Printing for patient-centred therapy. *Pharm. Res.* **2017**, *34*, 427–437. [CrossRef] [PubMed]

Proceeding Paper

A Protocol for the Evaluation of Nutritional and Functional Status Evolution During a Multidisciplinary Rehabilitation Program for Patients after SARS-CoV-2 Pneumonia [†]

Diogo Sousa-Catita [1,2,*], Catarina Godinho [1] and Jorge Fonseca [1,3]

1. PaMNEC—Grupo de Patologia Médica, Nutrição e Exercício Clínico, CiiEM—Centro de Investigação Interdisciplinar Egas Moniz, 2829-511 Almada, Portugal; cgodinho@egasmoniz.edu.pt (C.G.); jorgedafonseca@hotmail.com (J.F.)
2. Residências Montepio—Serviços de Saúde, SA, Sede—Rua Julieta Ferrão nº 10–5º, 1600-131 Lisboa, Portugal
3. GENE—Artificial Feeding Team, Gastroenterology Department, Hospital Garcia de Orta, 2805-267 Almada, Portugal
* Correspondence: diogo.rsc2@gmail.com
† Presented at the 5th International Congress of CiiEM—Reducing Inequalities in Health and Society, Online, 16–18 June 2021.

Abstract: Nutrition status is a major issue of the COVID-19 pandemic. Many factors associated with worse prognosis risk are related to nutrition. Patients received after hospital discharge for pneumonia due to SARS-Cov-2 were submitted to a multidisciplinary rehabilitation program. This study aimed to analyze the nutritional and functional status after SARS-Cov-2 pneumonia and evaluate the impact of a multidisciplinary rehabilitation program.

Keywords: SARS-CoV-2 pneumonia; nutritional and functional status; rehabilitation program

1. Introduction

Proper nutrition and good nutritional status have been gaining importance in the context of the COVID-19 pandemic. Food and nutrition are playing an important role in the prevention of disease and as one of the areas of priority intervention to minimize the consequences of this viral infection. Having a balanced diet contributes to a better nutritional status, an adequate immune response, decreases the risk of severe evolution and complications. Although the entire population is susceptible to SARS-CoV-2, most hospitalized patients are elderly and/or with nutrition-related chronic diseases (obesity, diabetes, hypertension, and cardiovascular diseases) [1]. All of these have the worst nutritional status, compromised immune system, and weakened respiratory system. The factors that have been associated with an increased risk of developing the severe COVID-19 disease and worse prognosis, such as hypoalbuminemia, lymphopenia, sarcopenia/fragility, high body mass index (BMI), and obesity, are related with malnutritional status [2]. Therefore, nutritional status plays an important role in COVID-19 being associated with a greater risk of developing severe illness and with a greater risk of hospitalization, ICU stay and death. On the other hand, patients who recovered from SARS-Cov-2 pneumonia present a decline in nutritional status, caused by the catabolic effect of the disease and by the hospital stay, with loss of muscle mass and function.

This study aimed to evaluate: (1) the nutritional and functional status of patients when they are received at the Residências Montepio (RM), transferred from hospitals after SARS-Cov-2 pneumonia; (2) the nutritional and functional status at the end of the rehabilitation program; and (3) the impact on the nutritional and functional status of the integrated and multidisciplinary rehabilitation program carried out after SARS-Cov-2 pneumonia. In addition, we intend to (4) assess food intake during the first 48 h of the rehabilitation program, because we suspect, from previous experience with these patients, that oral intake can be significantly reduced when compared with nutritional needs.

2. Materials and Methods

This is an observational, analytical, longitudinal study, evaluating no less than 110 adults. This will not have a pre-established duration, but it should not exceed 6 months. Statistical analysis will be used by SPSS to compare and correlate the nutritional and functional status variables, to see the nutritional and function impact of multidisciplinary rehabilitation program. The inclusion criteria are patients hospitalized in RM with a history of SARS-Cov-2 pneumonia agreeing to participate in the study and signing the informed consent. The exclusion criteria are patients with severe chronic underlying disorders that may clearly and very probably have a negative impact on the rehabilitation program. Each patient will only be part of the study while they are hospitalized in RM, from entrance (T0) until discharge (T2) 30 days later. At RM, they are submitted to an integrated and multidisciplinary rehabilitation program including 30 days of intensive rehabilitation, with physical therapy, occupational therapy, psychological intervention, speech therapy and personalized nutrition care, associated with medical and nursing care.

Each patient will be evaluated at three moments:
T0—Upon admission to the unit
T1—after 15 days
T2—Within 48 h before discharge
Each assessment will include the following parameters:

- Anthropometric data: weight, height, body mass index (BMI) according to age, geminal perimeter, brachial perimeter, tricipital skinfold (TSF), calculation of the muscular circumference of the arm.
- Functional assessment: hand grip strength assessed with pressure dynamometry.
- Scales: MNA [3]; GLIM and assessment of food intake in the first 24 h (24 h food recall) [4].
- Laboratory: routine blood count and serum albumin.

3. Results and Discussion

The present protocol was ratified by the Scientific Council of the Egas Moniz Higher School of Health and approved by the Ethics Committee (# 909). By 25 April, 107 patients aged 42–90 years were enrolled and 83 had already finished their protocols. We hope this protocol will show us if the different nutritional and function status in SARS-Cov-2 pneumonia patients has an influence on their recovery and future.

Institutional Review Board Statement: The study was conducted according to the guidelines of the Declaration of Helsinki, and approved by the Ethics Committee of Egas Moniz Higher School of Health (protocol code #909 of 17 December 2020).

Informed Consent Statement: Informed consent was obtained from all subjects involved in the study.

Data Availability Statement: Not applicable.

Acknowledgments: The authors declare no acknowledgments.

Conflicts of Interest: The authors declare no conflict of interest.

References

1. Aggarwal, S.; Garcia-Telles, N.; Aggarwal, G.; Lavie, C.; Lippi, G.; Henry, B.M. Clinical features, laboratory characteristics, and outcomes of patients hospitalized with coronavirus disease 2019 (COVID-19): Early report from the United States. *Diagnosis* **2020**, *7*, 91–96. [CrossRef] [PubMed]
2. Arentz, M.; Yim, E.; Klaff, L.; Lokhandwala, S.; Riedo, F.X.; Chong, M.; Lee, M. Characteristics and Outcomes of 21 Critically Ill Patients with COVID19 in Washington State. *JAMA* **2020**, *323*, 1612–1614. [CrossRef] [PubMed]

3. Kaiser, M.J.; Bauer, J.M.; Ramsch, C.; Uter, W.; Guigoz, Y.; Cederholm, T.; Thomas, D.R.; Anthony, P.; Charlton, K.E.; Maggio, M.; et al. Validation of the Mini Nutritional Assessment short-form (MNA®-SF): A practical tool for identification of nutritional status. *J. Nutr. Health Aging* **2009**, *13*, 782–788. [CrossRef]
4. Questionnaires from Nutrition Day (Sheet 2). Available online: https://www.nutritionday.org/cms/front_content.php?idart=477 (accessed on 11 December 2020).

Proceeding Paper

Tuning of Paroxetine 3D-Printable Formulations for Fused Deposition Modelling †

Sara Figueiredo [1], João F. Pinto [1], Fátima G. Carvalho [2] and Ana I. Fernandes [3,*]

1. iMed.ULisboa, Faculdade de Farmácia, Universidade de Lisboa, 1649-003 Lisboa, Portugal; sara.figueiredo@ff.ulisboa.pt (S.F.); jfpinto@ff.ul.pt (J.F.P.)
2. Infosaúde—Laboratório de Estudos Farmacêuticos, 2730-269 Barcarena, Portugal; fatimag.carvalho@anf.pt
3. CiiEM—Interdisciplinary Research Center Egas Moniz, Instituto Universitário Egas Moniz, 2829-511 Almada, Portugal
* Correspondence: aifernandes@egasmoniz.edu.pt; Tel.: +351-212946823
† Presented at the 5th International Congress of CiiEM—Reducing Inequalities in Health and Society, Online, 16–18 June 2021.

Abstract: This work reports the preliminary development of paroxetine-containing formulations amenable to hot-melt extrusion coupled to fused deposition modelling-based 3D printing. Polymeric matrices were used alone, or added with processing enhancers (e.g., plasticizer and filler). The polymeric formulation containing paroxetine (30% w/w), hydroxypropylcellulose (54% w/w) and excipients (16% w/w of dicalcium dihydrate phosphate, magnesium stearate and triethylcitrate; 10:1:5 ratio) exhibited the most suitable behaviour to be extruded and 3D printed, proving that adjuvants are critical to ensure processing of the formulations.

Keywords: extrudability; filament; printability; 3D-printed tablet; fused deposition modelling (FDM); hot melt extrusion (HME); paroxetine (PRX)

1. Introduction

Three-dimensional printing (3DP) has been the subject of an exponential interest in pharmacy by overcoming challenges of traditional manufacturing processes and allowing the production of patient-centric dosage forms [1]. Fused Deposition Modelling (FDM), the most widely used 3DP technique, requires the production of a drug-containing thermoplastic polymeric filament, obtained previously by hot-melt extrusion (HME), which is then melted and continuously deposited on a surface, layer by layer, building the 3D-printed dosage form [2].

The successful coupling of these two technologies depends on the concurrent extrudability of the raw materials and the printability of the filaments (FIL) obtained by HME, properties which are influenced by mechanical, rheological and thermal properties of materials [3]. Based on the selection of formulation and processing conditions, this work reports the preliminary development of 3D-printable formulations containing paroxetine (PRX) for HME coupled to FDM 3DP.

2. Materials and Methods

PRX (Lusifar, Lisbon, Portugal) was selected as a model drug; methylcellulose (MC) and hydroxypropylcellulose (HPC; HPC^{TM} LF and HPC^{TM} GF Pharm, Ashland Inc., Schaffhausen, Switzerland) and Soluplus® (SLP; Polyvinyl caprolactam-polyvinyl acetate-polyethylene glycol graft co-polymer, BASF, Ludwigshafen, Germany) were used as matrix-forming polymers. Dicalcium dihydrate phosphate (CaP) (Budenheim, Budenheim, Germany), magnesium stearate (MgSt) (Roic Pharma, Barcelona, Spain) and triethylcitrate (TEC) (Sigma Aldrich, Darmstadt, Germany) were used as adjuvants (F1-F8; see Table 1).

Table 1. Development and preliminary evaluation of PRX-based formulations regarding extrudability and printability in HME coupled to FDM 3D printing.

	Formulation Components (% w/w)								Extrudible [1] Temp. (°C)/Speed (rpm)	Printable [1] Temp. (°C)
	HPC GF	HPC LF	MC	SLP	CaP	MgSt	TEC	PRX		
F1	60	-	-	-	-	-	-	40	Yes (140/20)	No [2]
F3	-	-	-	60	-	-	-	40	Yes (160/20)	No [2]
F4	55	-	-	-	-	-	15	30	Yes (150/20)	No [3]
F5	-	55	-	-	-	-	15	30	Yes (150/20)	No [3]
F6	-	-	-	55	-	-	15	30	Yes (130/20)	No [3]
F7	54	-	-	-	10	1	5	30	Yes (120/10)	Yes (200/50)
F8	-	54	-	-	10	1	5	30	Yes (120/10)	Yes (200/50)

[1] Extrudability and printability represent the ability of the powder physical mixture and FIL to be successfully extruded and printable by HME and FDM 3DP, respectively. [2] High formulation viscosity and FIL too brittle. [3] FIL too pliable.

3D-printed tablets (TAB) containing PRX were prepared under the processing conditions described in Table 1, by combining HME (Notzek Pro single screw extruder, Notzek, Shoreham, UK) and FDM (3D printer Delta WASP 20 40 Turbo 2, Wasp, Massa Lombarda, Italy) technologies. Extrudability and printability of the different formulations were evaluated.

3. Results and Discussion

For the preliminary development of PRX-based formulations suitable for HME coupled to FDM 3DP, cellulose-derived polymers, such as MC (Tg = 184–197 °C) and HPC (Tg = 105 °C), and Soluplus® (Tg ≈ 70 °C) were selected [3]. The formulation containing MC (F2; Table 1) was the only unable to be extruded into FIL, since it requires higher temperature (>180 °C) and was thus excluded. The other polymers were successfully extruded by HME. Yet, these polymeric matrices generated non-printable FIL precluding FDM 3DP, due to surface irregularity and non-uniformity of diameter (closely related to the high viscosity of the formulation), thus preventing printer feeding. Mechanical properties of FIL proved to be inapt for 3DP since they were too brittle, rupturing inside the printing head, due to the forces applied by the extruding gear, which was ultimately responsible for blocking the printer.

3DP ability is directly influenced by the materials' properties [3] and processing conditions may be enhanced by addition of adjuvants. First, a plasticizer (TEC; 15% w/w) was used to reduce the polymer Tg and allow gentler HME temperature (F4-F6). Though obtained at lower temperatures, FIL were unable to be printed into TAB due to high ductility. Over-plasticization of the FIL caused permanent deformation along the printing head and feeding defects (mainly for F6, so SLP use was discontinued). To address this issue, TEC was decreased and replaced by the same amount of a filler (CaP). In turn, a small quantity of MgSt was added (F7-F8) to improve rheological properties of FIL. These HPC formulations were successfully extruded in PRX-loaded FIL apt to print TAB.

Fine tuning of formulations is proved crucial for optimal extrudability and printability.

Acknowledgments: This work was supported by the Fundação para a Ciência e a Tecnologia [grant number PTDC/CTM CTM/30949/2017 (Lisboa 010145 Feder 030949) and SFRH/BD/146968/2019].

Conflicts of Interest: The authors declare no conflict of interest.

References

1. Kolakovic, R.; Viitala, T.; Ihalainen, P.; Genina, N.; Peltonen, J.; Sandler, N. Printing technologies in fabrication of drug delivery systems. *Expert. Opin. Drug. Deliv.* **2013**, *10*, 1711–1725. [CrossRef]
2. Zhang, J.; Feng, X.; Patil, H.; Tiwari, R.V.; Repka, M.A. Coupling 3D printing with hot-melt extrusion to produce controlled-release tablets. *Int. J. Pharm.* **2017**, *519*, 186–197. [CrossRef] [PubMed]
3. Pereira, G.G.; Figueiredo, S.; Fernandes, A.I.; Pinto, J.F. Polymer selection for hot-melt extrusion coupled to fused deposition modelling in pharmaceutics. *Pharmaceutics* **2020**, *12*, 795. [CrossRef] [PubMed]

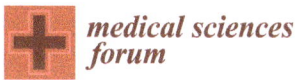

Proceeding Paper

Personality and Aggressive Behavior: The Relation between the Five-Factor and Aggression Models in a Domestic Violence Suspects Sample [†]

Ricardo Ventura Baúto [1,2,3,*], Ana Filipa Carreiro [3], Margarida Pereira [3], Renata Guarda [3] and Iris Almeida [1,2,3]

1. Instituto Universitário Egas Moniz (IUEM), Egas Moniz-Cooperativa de Ensino Superior, Crl., 2829-511 Almada, Portugal; ialmeida@egasmoniz.edu.pt
2. Laboratório de Psicologia (LabPSI), Centro de Investigação Interdisciplinar Egas Moniz (CiiEM), 2829-511 Almada, Portugal
3. Laboratório de Ciências Forenses e Psicológicas Egas Moniz (LCFPEM), 2829-511 Almada, Portugal; anafilipa205@gmail.com (A.F.C.); margarida.pereira96@hotmail.com (M.P.); renataguarda@live.com.pt (R.G.)
* Correspondence: rbauto.lcfpem@egasmoniz.edu.pt
† Presented at the 5th International Congress of CiiEM—Reducing Inequalities in Health and Society, Online, 16–18 June 2021.

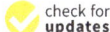

Citation: Baúto, R.V.; Carreiro, A.F.; Pereira, M.; Guarda, R.; Almeida, I. Personality and Aggressive Behavior: The Relation between the Five-Factor and Aggression Models in a Domestic Violence Suspects Sample. *Med. Sci. Forum* **2021**, *5*, 18. https://doi.org/10.3390/msf2021005018

Academic Editors: Helena Barroso and Cidália Castro

Published: 20 July 2021

Publisher's Note: MDPI stays neutral with regard to jurisdictional claims in published maps and institutional affiliations.

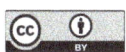

Copyright: © 2021 by the authors. Licensee MDPI, Basel, Switzerland. This article is an open access article distributed under the terms and conditions of the Creative Commons Attribution (CC BY) license (https://creativecommons.org/licenses/by/4.0/).

Abstract: The purpose of this study is to demonstrate the relationship between the five-factor model of personality and its association with aggression in 30 men and eight women who are suspects of domestic violence. The results show a positive correlation between neuroticism and hostility, a negative correlation between openness to experience and overall aggression, a negative correlation between agreeableness and physical aggression and anger, and a negative correlation between conscientiousness and anger. These results show us the need for personality assessment in domestic violence suspects and future research about personality and aggression.

Keywords: personality; aggressive behavior; five-factor model; domestic violence

1. Introduction

The five-factor model argues that personality is based on five core factors: neuroticism (calm, confident vs. anxious, pessimistic); extraversion (reserved, thoughtful vs. sociable, fun-loving); openness to experience (prefers routine, practical vs. imaginative, spontaneous); agreeableness (suspicious, uncooperative vs. trusting, helpful); and, finally, the conscientiousness (impulsive, disorganized vs. disciplined, careful) [1]. This model has been used to study offenses in general, antisocial behaviors, aggression, and violence [2]. Some studies [3–5] found that more neuroticism and less kindness and conscientiousness leads to problems related to antisocial personality and aggressive behaviors. Specifically, high neuroticism is associated with both increased aggression and mental distress in violent offenders [5].

2. Materials and Methods

The sample consisted of 38 suspects of domestic violence (n_{men} = 30 (78.9%); n_{women} = 8 (21.1%)), aged between 23 and 82 years old (M = 44.64, sd = 14.75) assessed in the Forensic Psychology Office of Forensic and Psychological Sciences Egas Moniz by Court and/or Public Prosecutor's Office. Most of the sample had middle school education (66.7% (n = 21)) and had mostly unqualified jobs (26.3% (n = 10)) or were unemployed (21.2% (n = 8)). Most individuals were single (52.8%), forward by married (25%) and divorced (22.5%). Regarding the relationship between our sample and their victims, a large proportion was ex-partners (36.8%). Regarding criminal history, 65.8% (n = 25) had previous contacts with the Justice System, including convictions in 39.5% (n = 15) of cases.

Data were collected from lawsuits, semi-structured interviews, collateral information, and clinical and forensic assessment tools (e.g., NEO-PI-R; BPAQ).

3. Results and Discussion

The results show that suspects of domestic violence have moderate neuroticism ($M = 61.21$; $sd = 25.24$). In the aggression assessment, the results show that domestic violence suspects had a greater tendency for hostility ($M = 18.23$; $sd = 30.05$). Table 1 shows the correlations between the five-factor model (NEO-PI-R) and aggression (BPAQ). The results show us a positive correlation between neuroticism and hostility, a negative correlation between openness to experience and overall aggression, a negative correlation between agreeableness and physical aggression and anger, and a negative correlation between conscientiousness and anger.

Table 1. Relationship between personality and aggression.

	Neuroticism	Openness to Experience	Agreeableness	Conscientiousness
Physical aggression	−0.318	−0.479	−0.611 **	−0.319
Anger	−0.138	−0.380	−0.624 **	−0.559 *
Hostility	0.601 *	−0.410	−0.129	−0.240
Total agression	0.019	−0.487 *	−0.570 *	−0.427

** $p < 0.01$; * $p < 0.05$.

Results are discussed in terms of why personality should be considered in assessments of domestic violence suspects, and for that purpose, it is necessary for future research to be conducted. These results show us the need for personality assessment in domestic violence suspects and the need for a reasonable articulation in Forensic Psychology and Law.

Institutional Review Board Statement: This study is part of a protocol established among the Portuguese Public Prosecutor's Office and Egas Moniz - Higher Education School to assess and analyze the characteristics of victims and offenders in the field of Violence. The strictness of ethical and deontological principles are safeguarded once criminal records have been restricted access by law (including judicial secrecy). Therefore, all assessed subjects gave their informed consent, and their data were processed anonymously.

Informed Consent Statement: All ethical issues were considered due to the sensitive nature of the detailed data, the respective informed consent, confidentiality limits, and information about the ethics and technician's impartiality.

Data Availability Statement: Data sharing not applicable because part of information derives from criminal records.

Conflicts of Interest: The authors declare no conflict of interest.

References

1. Costa, P.; McCrae, R. *NEO-PI-R: Manual Profissional*; Cegoc-Tea: Lisboa, Portugal, 2000.
2. Becerra-García, J.A.; García-León, A.; Muela-Martinez, J.A.; Egan, V. A controlled study of the Big Five personality dimensions in sex offenders, non-sex offenders and non-offenders: Relationship with offending behaviour and childhood abuse. *J. Forensic Psychiatry Psychol.* **2013**, *24*, 233–246. [CrossRef]
3. Miller, J.D.; Lynam, D.R.; Jones, S. Externalizing behaviour through the lens of the Fiver-Factor Model: A focus on agreeableness and conscientiousness. *J. Personal. Assess.* **2008**, *90*, 158–164. [CrossRef] [PubMed]
4. Blackburn, R.; Renwick, S.D.; Donnelly, J.P.; Logan, C. Big five or big two? Superordinate factors in the NEO Five-Factor Inventory and the Antisocial Personality Questionnaire. *Personal. Individ. Differ.* **2004**, *37*, 957–970. [CrossRef]
5. Jones, S.E.; Miller, J.D.; Lynam, D.R. Personality, antisocial behaviour, and aggression: A meta-analytic review. *J. Crim. Justice* **2011**, *39*, 329–337. [CrossRef]

Proceeding Paper

Characterization of CYP2C19*17 Polymorphism in a Portuguese Population Sample Relevant for Proton Pump Inhibitor Therapy—A Pilot Study [†]

Adriana M. L. Ferraz [1], Susana Bandarra [1], Paulo Mascarenhas [1], Isabel Barahona [1], Rui Martins [2] and Ana Clara Ribeiro [1,*]

[1] Laboratoório de Biologia Molecular, Centro de Investigacão Interdisciplinar Egas Moniz (CiiEM), Instituto Universitário Egas Moniz (IUEM), 2829-511 Caparica, Portugal; adrianamlferraz@gmail.com (A.M.L.F.); sbandarra@egasmoniz.edu.pt (S.B.); pmascarenhas@egasmoniz.edu.pt (P.M.); ibarahona@egasmoniz.edu.pt (I.B.)

[2] Faculdade de Ciências, Centro de Estatística e Aplicações—Universidade de Lisboa, 1749-016 Lisbon, Portugal; ruimartins@ymail.com

* Correspondence: acribeiro@egasmoniz.edu.pt

[†] Presented at the 5th International Congress of CiiEM—Reducing inequalities in Health and Society, Online, 16–18 June 2021.

Abstract: The interindividual variability of Proton Pump Inhibitor (PPI) therapy results from the phenotype variability associated with the cytochrome P450 2C19 (CYP2C19) gene, namely the CYP2C19*17 allele. Our aim was to characterize patients' genetic variability undergoing PPI therapy. A sample of 33 oral mucosa cells from Portuguese pharmacy patients was collected, followed by genotyping. The allelic frequencies of CYP2C19*1 (-806C) and CYP2C19*17 (-806T) were 71.2% and 28.8%, respectively. The genotypic frequencies for CYP2C19*1/*1 and CYP2C19*1/*17 were 42.4% and 57.6%, respectively, and 19 of these patients may have a Rapid Metabolizer (RM) phenotype pharmaceutical opinion letter, based on genetic evidence.

Keywords: cytochrome P450 2C19; pharmacogenetics; proton pump inhibitors

1. Introduction

The genotypic variability associated with the CYP2C19 gene is the pharmacogenetic factor (PGx) that predominantly affects the therapeutic response to PPIs [1]. The CYP2C19*17 polymorphism (-806C>T) results in the replacement of a cytosine (C) with a thymine (T) at -806 nucleotide position in the promoter region of the CYP2C19 gene [2]. The CYP2C19*17 variant is associated with increased enzyme activity, so the monitoring of patients should be considered in terms of therapeutic failure risk [1,2]. The future of PGx in clinical practice may be at the origin of its implementation at community Portuguese pharmacies. In this sense, the present study intends to characterize the genotypic and phenotypic variability of the CYP2C19*17 polymorphism in order to develop a strategy focused and oriented for the Portuguese population.

2. Materials and Methods

The analyzed sample corresponds to a total of 33 patients receiving therapy with PPIs at Nobre Guerreiro community pharmacy (Seixal, Portugal); inclusion criteria: over-the-counter PPI therapy prescribed in Portugal; exclusion criteria: <18 y.o. without cognitive deficits or language barriers preventing information collection. This study was previously approved by the Ethics Committee of Egas Moniz (EM). DNA extraction was performed according to the manufacturer's instructions from the commercial kit QIAamp®. Genotyping was performed using PCR-RFLP. The oligonucleotide primers used for the amplification of CYP2C19*17 were forward 5′-GCCCTTAGCACCAAATTCTC-3′ and reverse

5′-ATTTAACCCCCTAAAAAAACACG-3′ primers [2]. PCR products were digested with *Sfa*NI restriction endonuclease. For the CYP2C19*17 polymorphism, the wild-type (wt) genotype CYP2C19*1/*1 (-806C/C, 184bp, 139bp and 114bp) and the heterozygous genotype CYP2C19*1/*17 (-806C/T, 218bp, 184bp, 139bp and 114bp) [1,2] were documented. PCR products were purified and sequenced in both DNA directions. The nucleotide sequences were analyzed with BioEdit Alignment Editor V.7.2.5. The statistical analysis was performed using R Statistical software v. 4.0 (Free Software Foundation, Boston, MA, USA) based on the chi-square test (χ^2) and a 95% confidence level. Results were compared with those expected for a population in the Hardy–Weinberg (H-W) equilibrium.

3. Results and Discussion

In the population studied (21 females and 12 males; 17 Caucasians and 16 Africans, in the age range between 21 and 89 y.o.), the CYP2C19*17 polymorphism is not in H-W equilibrium ($p < 0.05$). There are no significant differences between ethnicities and genders in allelic and genotypic frequencies ($p > 0.05$). Caucasian patients represented a genotypic frequency of 12.1% for CYP2C19*1/*17 (-806C/T) and Negroid patients had a genotype frequency of 36.4%. The female gender had a genotypic frequency of 33.3% for the genotype CYP2C19*1/*17 (-806C/T) and the male gender represented the genotypic frequency of 24.2%. In the present study, 19 patients have the CYP2C19*1/*17 genotype (-806C/T) associated with the RM phenotype. In these patients, it is necessary to increase the dose to prevent therapeutic failure. The CYP2C19*1/*17 genotype (-806C/T) and the respective RM phenotype were found in the European population (36%) [1], as well as in the present sample (57.6%). The CYP2C19*17 allele demonstrated a frequency in Germany (25.5%), Norway (22.0%) and Sweden (20.0%) [3] similar to the allelic frequency herein obtained (28.8%) (Table 1).

Table 1. Comparison of allelic frequencies of CYP2C19 reported from different populations. Data adapted from 1000 Genomes Project [3] and those obtained in the sample under study.

Country	N	CYP2C19*1 (%)	CYP2C19*17 (%)
Portugal	33	71.2	28.8
Norway	309	62.8	22.0
Spain	346	75.0	10.0
Germany	186	59.3	25.5
Sweden	185	64.0	20.0

In conclusion, the implementation of a PGx service is an imperative need for the success of PPI therapy, considering the variability of the CYP2C19 gene and the increasing use of PPIs in recent years, to ensure the success of PPI therapy in Portugal.

Institutional Review Board Statement: The study was conducted according to the guidelines of the Declaration of Helsinki, and approved by the Ethics Committee of Egas Moniz (No. 817 of 29 September 2020).

Informed Consent Statement: Informed consent was obtained from all subjects involved in the study.

Data Availability Statement: The data presented in this study are available on request from the corresponding author.

Acknowledgments: Nobre Guerreiro community pharmacy (Amora, Portugal) and the Health Centre of Amora. This work was part of Adriana Ferraz's master degree in Pharmaceutical Sciences and it was supported by EM.

Conflicts of Interest: The authors declare no conflict of interest.

References

1. Lima, J.J.; Thomas, C.D.; Barbarino, J.; Desta, Z.; Van Driest, S.L.; El Rouby, N.; Johnson, J.A.; Cavallari, L.H.; Shakhnovich, V.; Thacker, D.L.; et al. Clinical pharmacogenetics implementation consortium (CPIC) guideline for CYP2C19 and proton pump inhibitor dosing. *Clin. Pharmacol. Ther.* **2020**, *109*, 1417–1423. [CrossRef] [PubMed]
2. Dehbozorgi, M.; Kamalidehghan, B.; Hosseini, I.; Dehghanfard, Z.; Sangtarash, M.H.; Firoozi, M.; Ahmadipour, F.; Meng, G.Y.; Houshmand, M. Prevalence of the CYP2C19*2 (681 G>A), *3 (636 G>A) and *17 (-806 C>T) alleles among an Iranian population of different ethnicities. *Mol. Med. Rep.* **2018**, *17*, 4195–4202. [CrossRef] [PubMed]
3. International Genome Sample Resource. 1000 Genomes Project. Available online: https://www.internationalgenome.org (accessed on 10 December 2020).

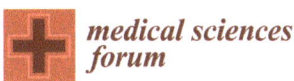

Proceeding Paper

Mouth Breathing and Atypical Swallowing in Adult Orthodontic Patients at Egas Moniz Dental Clinic: A Pilot Study [†]

Ana Raquel Barata [1,2,*], Gunel Kizi [1,2], Luis Proença [1], Valter Alves [2] and Ana Sintra Delgado [1,2]

1. Centro de Investigação Interdisciplinar Egas Moniz (CiiEM), Egas Moniz Cooperativa de Ensino Superior, C.R.L., 2829-511 Almada, Portugal; gunelkizi@outlook.com (G.K.); lproenca@egasmoniz.edu.pt (L.P.); anasintradelgado@gmail.com (A.S.D.)
2. Consulta Assistencial de Ortodontia, Clínica Dentária Egas Moniz, Egas Moniz Cooperativa de Ensino Superior, C.R.L., 2829-511 Almada, Portugal; valtervpa@hotmail.com
* Correspondence: raquelgarciabarata@gmail.com; Tel.: +351-918781723
† Presented at the 5th International Congress of CiiEM—Reducing Inequalities in Health and Society, Online, 16–18 June 2021.

Abstract: Background: Mouth breathing and atypical swallowing are myofunctional problems, emerging as a pathological adaptation. This exploratory study was aimed to investigate the possible relation between breathing and swallowing patterns in adults. Methods: A total of 58 patients referred to the Orthodontic Department at Egas Moniz Dental Clinic were enrolled. Results: Atypical swallowing was more prevalent in women (78.0%) than in men (47.1%). A significantly higher proportion of patients exhibiting both mouth breathing and atypical swallowing were identified (46.6%). Swallowing pattern was found to be significantly associated with gender and breathing pattern.

Keywords: mouth-breathing; atypical swallowing; myofunctional problems; adults

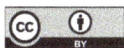

1. Introduction

Physiological swallowing and breathing are often affected by anatomic or functional problems [1,2]. Most breathing is nasal, and mouth breathing can be thought of like a pathological adaptation, as it can lead to a series of changes that are often irreversible for the growth and development of a child [3]. Atypical swallowing is a functional problem that consists in an altered tongue position during the act of swallowing [4]. The high incidence in population, multifactorial etiology, and the recurring connection with the presence of malocclusions made it a topic of strong interest in the literature. Mouth breathing and atypical swallowing are myofunctional problems that can be found, emerging as a pathological adaptation, that often produce irreversible changes in growth and development [5,6]. This study was aimed to investigate the possible relation between breathing and swallowing patterns in adults.

2. Materials and Methods

A total of 58 patients—41 females (70.7%) and 17 males (29.3%)—referred to the of Orthodontic Department at Egas Moniz Dental Clinic (EMDC) between January 2018 and February 2019, participated in this study. The study was approved by the Ethics Committee of Egas Moniz. Inclusion criteria were being adult with no previous orthodontic treatment or craniofacial anomalies, having a clinical record at EMDC, along with the correspondent informed consent signed. The method used to assess breathing and swallowing patterns was adapted by Marchesan [7]. Data were analyzed by using descriptive and inferential methodologies. A significance level of 5% was set in the latter case.

3. Results and Discussion

A relatively high prevalence of patients exhibiting both mouth breathing and atypical swallowing (n = 27, 46.6% from total) was observed (Table 1). However, the value was inferior to the one reported in a similar study (97.2%) [8]. A higher prevalence of mouth-breathers was found in women (n = 23, 56.1%) than in men (n = 7, 41.2%). Atypical swallowing was also more prevalent in women (n = 32, 78.0%) than in men (n = 8, 47.1%). Conversely to what was found in the study by Maspero et al. [2], the association between breathing pattern and swallowing pattern was found to be significant (p < 0.001). Moreover, swallowing pattern was found to be significantly associated with gender (p = 0.020). Further studies are mandatory to clarify these findings.

Table 1. Distribution of breathing and swallowing patterns, presented as n (% from total M | F).

		Swallowing		
		Correct	Incorrect	Total
		M	F	M	F	M	F
Breathing	Nasal	7 (70.0)	8 (44.4)	3 (30.0)	10 (55.6)	10	18
	Oral	2 (28.6)	1 (4.3)	5 (71.4)	22 (95.7)	7	23
	Total	9 (52.9)	9 (22.0)	8 (47.1)	32 (78.0)	17	41

Institutional Review Board Statement: The study was conducted according to the guidelines of the Declaration of Helsinki, and approved by the Ethics Committee of Egas Moniz Higher Education Cooperative (protocol code 600).

Informed Consent Statement: Informed consent was obtained from all subjects involved in the study. Written informed consent has been obtained from the patient(s) to publish this paper.

Data Availability Statement: MDPI Research Data Policies.

Conflicts of Interest: The authors declare no conflict of interest.

References

1. Chambi-Rocha, A.; Cabrera-Domínguez, M.E.; Domínguez-Reyes, A. Breathing mode influence on craniofacial development and head posture. *J. Pediatria* **2018**, *94*, 123–130. [CrossRef] [PubMed]
2. Maspero, C.; Prevedello, C.; Giannini, L.; Galbiati, G.; Farronato, G. Atypical swallowing: A review. *Minerva Stomatol.* **2014**, *63*, 217–227. [PubMed]
3. Matsuo, K.; Palmer, J.B. Coordination of Mastication, Swallowing and Breathing. *Jpn. Dent. Sci. Rev.* **2009**, *45*, 31–40. [CrossRef] [PubMed]
4. Yamaguchi, S.; Ishida, M.; Hidaka, K.; Gomi, S.; Takayama, S.; Sato, K.; Yoshioka, Y.; Wakayama, N.; Sekine, K.; Matsune, S.; et al. Relationship between swallowing function and breathing/phonation. *Nasus Larynx* **2018**, *45*, 533–539. [CrossRef] [PubMed]
5. Di Vecchio, S.; Manzini, P.; Candida, E.; Gargari, M. Froggy mouth: A new myofunctional approach to atypical swallowing. *Eur. J. Paediatr. Dent.* **2019**, *20*, 33–37. [CrossRef] [PubMed]
6. Ambrosio, A.R.; Trevillatto, P.C.; Sakima, T.; Ignácio, S.A.; Shimizu, R.H. Correlation between morphology and function of the upper lip: A longitudinal evaluation. *Eur. J. Orthod.* **2009**, *31*, 306–313. [CrossRef] [PubMed]
7. Andrade, F.; Araújo, A.; Ribeiro, C.; Deccax, L.; Nemr, K. Alterações estruturais de órgãos fonoarticulares e más oclusões dentárias em respiradores orais de 6 a 10 anos. *Respiração Oral Sist. Estomatognático Ver.* **2005**, *7*, 318–325.
8. Lemos, C.; Junqueira, P.; Gomez, M.; Faria, M.; Basso, S. Study of the relationship between the dentition and the swallowing of mouth breathers. *Int. Otorrinolaringol.* **2006**, *10*, 114–118.

Proceeding Paper

Exploring Inequalities in HPV Vaccine Uptake among Cape Verdean Immigrant and Portuguese Native Women [†]

Violeta Alarcão [1,2,*], Pedro Candeias [2], Sónia Pintassilgo [1] and Fernando Luís Machado [1]

1. Centro de Investigação e Estudos de Sociologia, Iscte-Instituto Universitário de Lisboa, Avenida das Forças Armadas, 1649-026 Lisboa, Portugal; sonia.cardoso@iscte-iul.pt (S.P.); fernando.machado@iscte-iul.pt (F.L.M.)
2. Instituto de Saúde Ambiental, Faculdade de Medicina, Universidade de Lisboa, Avenida Professor Egas Moniz, 1649-028 Lisboa, Portugal; pedromecandeias@gmail.com
* Correspondence: violeta_sabina_alarcao@iscte-iul.pt
† Presented at the 5th International Congress of CiiEM—Reducing inequalities in Health and Society, Online, 16–18 June 2021.

Abstract: Based on data from the FEMINA study, this communication aims to explore inequalities in HPV vaccine uptake. Results highlighted differences between the Portuguese and the Cape Verdean women: 97% vs. 67% had heard about the HPV vaccine; 30% vs. 9% had been vaccinated, and 71% vs. 82% had reported a lack of medical recommendation as a major reason for not having been vaccinated. Further research on the mechanisms that operate in the production of health disparities is needed to promote equity-focused interventions.

Keywords: HPV vaccination; sexual health; health disparities; ethnicity

1. Introduction

The sociological understanding of the human papillomavirus (HPV) vaccination offers the possibility to better understand society, because the discourses on HPV vaccination are also about sexuality, gender, power, and identity. Social science research has pointed to the shifting processes by which individuals receive and accept medical definitions and interventions on their bodies, including professional claims of knowledge and increasing focus on risk mitigation through personal behavior [1–3]. Trust in one's doctor, in the healthcare system, and in the pharmaceutical industry are also part of this process that shapes health-related beliefs and influences HPV vaccine decision-making [4]. The Portuguese National Health System (NHS) is responsible for implementing the National Immunization Program in Portugal. People can be vaccinated in local primary healthcare centers, and vaccines that are included in the program are free for all NHS users. High levels of immunization are achieved in Portugal, including against HPV. However, information is missing regarding vaccination coverage among racial and ethnic groups.

2. Materials and Methods

Between March and September 2020, a cross-sectional computer-assisted telephone interviewing survey was conducted among a probabilistic sample of Cape Verdean immigrant and Portuguese native adult women residents in the Metropolitan Area of Lisbon. Survey design and data collection have previously been detailed [5]. The inclusion criteria included: (a) age—between 18 and 49 years; (b) born in Portugal or in Cape Verde; (c) both parents born in Portugal (for those born in Portugal) or both parents born in Cape Verde (for those born in Cape Verde); and (d) able to give informed consent to participate in the research. Participants were asked if they had been vaccinated or not and the multiple possible reasons for having been vaccinated or not having been vaccinated (list of different motives and possibility of indicating other non-listed motives).

3. Results and Discussion

Cape Verdean women (n = 151) were younger (43.7% vs. 24.5% aged less than 30, $p < 0.001$) than the Portuguese women (n = 102), and their mothers had a lower educational level (64.9% vs. 35.5% with an education until the fourth grade, $p < 0.001$). Around 58% of the Cape Verdean women who had arrived in Portugal were aged more than 18. The results highlighted differences between Portuguese and Cape Verdean women regarding HPV knowledge (97% vs. 67% had heard about the HPV vaccine), HPV vaccine uptake (30% vs. 9% had been vaccinated), and underlying motives for both being vaccinated and not being vaccinated (71% vs. 82% had reported a lack of medical recommendation as a major reason for not having been vaccinated). Table 1 shows the distribution of HPV vaccine uptake and associated factors. Besides younger age and (higher) mothers' educational level, being a Portuguese native woman was a strong predictor for HPV vaccine uptake (aOR = 8.877, $p < 0.001$).

Table 1. HPV vaccine uptake and associated factors.

	HPV Vaccine Uptake	No HPV Vaccine Uptake	Crude OR * (p Value)	Model 1 ** Adjusted OR (p Value) Nagelkerke Pseudo R^2 = 0.220	Model 2 *** Adjusted OR (p Value) Nagelkerke Pseudo R^2 = 0.462
Age (years), mean	26.82	35.33	0.879 (<0.001)	0.890 (<0.001)	0.843 (<0.001)
Mothers' educational level,%					
Until fourth grade	5.97	94.03	1.00	1.00	1.00
Higher than the fourth grade	31.09	68.91	7.107 (<0.001)	6.371 (<0.001)	3.606 (=0.012)
Age at first intercourse (years), mean	16.83	17.65	0.840 (=0.041)	0.869 (=0.184)	0.928 (=0.479)
Country of birth, %					
Portugal	30.4	69.6	4.273 (<0.001)		8.877 (<0.001)
Cape Verde	9.3	90.7	1.00		1.00

* Odds ratio (ORs) were computed by comparing HPV vaccine uptake vs. no HPV vaccine uptake in logistic regression models; ** Model 1 is adjusted for age, mothers' educational level, and age at first intercourse; *** Model 2 is adjusted to all variables.

This was a small-scale study, designed to explore sexual and reproductive health in general and not specifically focused on HPV vaccination. Therefore, these exploratory findings on the HPV vaccine uptake are not generalizable for the Portuguese population or for migrant populations in Portugal. This study highlights health inequalities in Portugal between the Cape Verdean immigrant population (one of the oldest and most represented foreign populations) and the autochthonous population. Considering that some immigrants arrive after the recommend age for HPV vaccination, health professionals are recommended to adapt the HPV communication to immigrant families, in particular those from countries with no HPV vaccine coverage reported [6].

Funding: The FEMINA project (PTDC/SOC-SOC/30025/2017) was granted by FCT.

Institutional Review Board Statement: The study was conducted according to the guidelines of the Declaration of Helsinki, and approved by the Ethics Committee of the Centro Académico de Medicina de Lisboa (466/18 approved on 14 May 2019).

Informed Consent Statement: Informed consent was obtained from all subjects involved in the study.

Data Availability Statement: To protect the confidentiality of research participants, data are not publicly available.

Conflicts of Interest: The authors declare no conflict of interest.

References

1. Clarke, A.; Shim, J.; Mamo, L.; Fosket, J.; Fishman, J. Biomedicalization: Technoscientific Transformations of Health, Illness, and U.S. Biomedicine. *Am. Sociol. Rev.* **2003**, *68*, 161–194. [CrossRef]
2. Siu, J.Y.M.; Fung, T.K.F.; Leung, L.H.M. Social and cultural construction processes involved in HPV vaccine hesitancy among Chinese women: A qualitative study. *Int. J. Equity Health* **2019**, *18*, 1–18. [CrossRef] [PubMed]

3. Reich, J.A. Vaccine Refusal and Pharmaceutical Acquiescence: Parental Controland Ambivalence in Managing Children's Health. *Am. Sociol. Rev.* **2020**, *85*, 106–127. [CrossRef]
4. MacArthur, K.R. Beyond health beliefs: The role of trust in the HPV vaccine decision-making process among American college students. *Health Sociol. Rev.* **2017**, *26*, 321–338. [CrossRef]
5. Alarcão, V.; Stefanovska-Petkovska, M.; Virgolino, A.; Santos, O.; Ribeiro, S.; Costa, A.; Nogueira, P.; Pascoal, P.M.; Pintassilgo, S.; Machado, F.L. Fertility, Migration and Acculturation (FEMINA): A research protocol for studying intersectional sexual and reproductive health inequalities. *Reprod. Health* **2019**, *16*, 140. [CrossRef]
6. Bruni, L.; Saura-Lázaro, A.; Montoliu, A.; Brotons, M.; Alemany, L.; Diallo, M.S.; Afsard, O.Z.; LaMontagne, D.S.; Mosina, L.; Contreras, M.; et al. HPV vaccination introduction worldwide and WHO and UNICEF estimates of national HPV immunization coverage 2010–2019. *Prev. Med.* **2021**, *144*, 106399. [CrossRef]

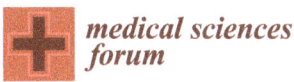

Proceeding Paper

Treatment of Patients with Somatic Tinnitus Attributed to Temporomandibular Disorder: A Case Report †

Paula Moleirinho-Alves [1,2,*], Pedro Cebola [1,3], André Almeida [1,2,3], Haúla Haider [1] and João Paço [1]

1. Cuf Tejo Hospital, 1350-352 Lisboa, Portugal; pedro.cebola@cuf.pt (P.C.); andre.mariz.almeida@cuf.pt (A.A.); haula.f.haider@cuf.pt (H.H.); joao.paco@cuf.pt (J.P.)
2. PaMNEC—Grupo de Patologia Médica, Nutrição e Exercício Clínico, CiiEM—Centro de Investigação Interdisciplinar Egas Moniz, 2829-511 Almada, Portugal
3. Egas Moniz Higher Institute of Health Science, 2829-511 Almada, Portugal
* Correspondence: paula.m.alves@cuf.pt; Tel.: +351-966-457-961
† Presented at the 5th International Congress of CiiEM—Reducing inequalities in Health and Society, Online, 16–18 June 2021.

Abstract: Tinnitus is a common symptom described in patients with temporomandibular disorders (TMDs), affecting quality of life and frequently causing distress. Somatic or somatosensory tinnitus can be attributed to the somatic system of the temporomandibular or cervical spine. Due to the multifactorial etiology of TMD, its management should be based on a multidisciplinary approach. Dentists and physical therapists may play a role in the individual and multimodal management of such patients. The aim of this case study is to analyse the effects of the conservative multidisciplinary management of tinnitus in patients with coexisting tinnitus, TMD and bruxism.

Keywords: tinnitus; TMD; dentists; physiotherapy; otolaryngologist; multidisciplinary team

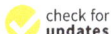

Citation: Moleirinho-Alves, P.; Cebola, P.; Almeida, A.; Haider, H.; Paço, J. Treatment of Patients with Somatic Tinnitus Attributed to Temporomandibular Disorder: A Case Report. *Med. Sci. Forum* **2021**, *5*, 22. https://doi.org/10.3390/msf2021005022

Academic Editors: Helena Barroso and Cidália Castro

Published: 21 July 2021

Publisher's Note: MDPI stays neutral with regard to jurisdictional claims in published maps and institutional affiliations.

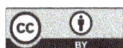

Copyright: © 2021 by the authors. Licensee MDPI, Basel, Switzerland. This article is an open access article distributed under the terms and conditions of the Creative Commons Attribution (CC BY) license (https://creativecommons.org/licenses/by/4.0/).

1. Introduction

Temporomandibular disorders (TMDs) present a range of signs and symptoms, which include pain in the masticatory muscles and joints and limitations in the range of mandibular movement. However, patients with TMD may also have other associated symptoms, especially otological symptoms such as tinnitus [1]. The definition of tinnitus can be described as the conscious perception of and the reaction to a sound in the absence of a corresponding external acoustic stimulus, commonly described as a "phantom" perception. It is considered to be a symptom and not a disease in itself [2]. Its etiology is multifactorial and, in addition to hearing loss or sound trauma, it can also be associated with the somatic system of the cervical spine or temporomandibular area, namely the temporomandibular joint (TMJ) and/or chewing muscles. This tinnitus is called somatic or somatosensory and has been described in 36–43% of a population with subjective tinnitus. The frequent coexistence of tinnitus and temporomandibular disorders (TMD) has already been demonstrated in scientific literature [3]. A recent review reported that the prevalence of tinnitus is higher in patients with TMD (35.8% to 60.7%) when compared to patients without TMD (9.7% to 26.0%) with an odds ratio of 4.45 [1]. The aim of this case study is to analyze the effects of conservative multidisciplinary management of tinnitus in patients with coexisting tinnitus, TMD and bruxism.

2. Materials and Methods

A 27-year-old male patient with tinnitus and myalgia in the masticatory muscles self-reported awake and sleep bruxism. The patient was initially evaluated by an otolaryngologist and the patient can positively correlate the beginning of the manifestation of the painful symptoms with tinnitus. Pain intensity is measured with a numeric pain rating scale (NPRS) and tinnitus is assessed with the Tinnitus Handicap Inventory (THI).

The Tinnitus Handicap Inventory is a reliable and valid questionnaire to evaluate tinnitus-related disability in patients with tinnitus. The THI consists of 25 items. In the THI, scores of 0, 2, or 4 are assigned to each answer, and thus the total score ranges from 0 to 100. Higher THI scores indicate a greater handicap from tinnitus, and five categories are used: no handicap (0–16), mild handicap (18–36), moderate handicap (38–56), severe handicap (58–76), and catastrophic handicap (78–100) [4]. The Portuguese version of the THI total has a very good internal consistency with a Cronbach's alpha coefficient of 0.86 [5]. The treatment plan consisted of cognitive-behavioural therapy with a first appointment based on education and habit recognition and modification, and the patient was medicated with muscle relaxants, provided with an occlusal stabilization splint, and performed stretching techniques and therapeutic exercises. All the assumptions of the Helsinki Declaration have been fulfilled and informed consent was approved by the ethics commission of Egas Moniz Higher Institute of Health Science (process number 675).

3. Results and Discussion

During the initial assessment, the NPRS of the left masseter was seven and that of the left temporalis was four. The THI score was 42, which indicated a moderate handicap. Four weeks after the beginning of the treatment plan, the patient referred to the absence of tinnitus and myalgia in the masticatory muscles and a greater awareness of awake bruxism. These findings are in agreement with those verified by other authors and suggest that the approaches for patients with somatic tinnitus should be multimodal [6]. In patients with tinnitus, as well as TMD or bruxism, improvement in tinnitus seems to be achieved by controlling TMJ complaints [3]. It is necessary to use the best available TMD treatment option to gain maximal improvement in tinnitus complaints. Multimodal therapies seem to be an appropriate approach for these patients.

Institutional Review Board Statement: The study was conducted according to the guidelines of the Declaration of Helsinki, and approved by the Institutional Review Board (or Ethics Committee) of Egas Moniz Higher Institute of Health Science (protocol code 675, 13 February 2019).

Informed Consent Statement: Informed consent was obtained from all subjects involved in the study.

Conflicts of Interest: The authors declare no conflict of interest.

References

1. Plaza-Manzano, G.; Delgado-de-la-Serna, P.; Díaz-Arribas, M.J.; Rodrigues-de-Souza, D.P.; Fernández-de-Las-Peñas, C.; Alburquerque-Sendín, F. Influence of Clinical, Physical, Psychological, and Psychophysical Variables on Treatment Outcomes in Somatic Tinnitus Associated with Temporomandibular Pain: Evidence From a Randomized Clinical Trial. *Pain Pract.* **2021**, *21*, 8–17. [CrossRef] [PubMed]
2. Haider, H.F.; Hoare, D.J.; Costa, R.F.P.; Potgieter, I.; Kikidis, D.; Lapira, A.; Nikitas, C.; Caria, H.; Cunha, N.T.; Paço, J.C. Pathophysiology, Diagnosis and Treatment of Somatosensory Tinnitus: A Scoping Review. *Front. Neurosci.* **2017**, *11*, 207. [CrossRef] [PubMed]
3. Michiels, S.; van der Wal, A.C.; Nieste, E.; Van de Heyning, P.; Braem, M.; Visscher, C.; Topsakal, V.; Gilles, A.; Jacquemin, L.; Hesters, M.; et al. Conservative therapy for the treatment of patients with somatic tinnitus attributed to temporomandibular dysfunction: Study protocol of a randomised controlled trial. *Trials* **2018**, *19*, 554. [CrossRef] [PubMed]
4. Wakabayashi, S.; Oishi, N.; Shinden, S.; Ogawa, K. Factor analysis and evaluation of each item of the tinnitus handicap inventory. *Head Face Med.* **2020**, *16*, 4. [CrossRef] [PubMed]
5. Oliveira, V.; Menezes, R.F. Avaliação da incapacidade resultante dos zumbidos: Versão portuguesa do Tinnitus Handicap Inventory (THI). In *Livro de Resumos da XI Conferência Internacional de Avaliação Psicológica: Formas e Contextos*; Psiquilíbrios: Braga, Portugal, 2006; p. 30.
6. Serna, P.D.; Plaza-Manzano, G.; Cleland, J.; Fernández-de-las-Peñas, C.; Martín-Casas, P.; Díaz-Arribas, M. Effects of Cervico-Mandibular Manual Therapy in Patients with Temporomandibular Pain Disorders and Associated Somatic Tinnitus: A Randomized Clinical Trial. *Pain Med.* **2020**, *21*, 613–624. [CrossRef] [PubMed]

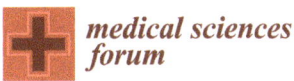

Proceeding Paper

Incidence of Oral Mucositis in Patients Undergoing Head and Neck Cancer Treatment: Systematic Review and Meta-Analysis [†]

Raquel Pacheco [1,*], Maria Alzira Cavacas [1], Paulo Mascarenhas [1], Pedro Oliveira [1,2] and Carlos Zagalo [1]

1. CiiEM Morphology Lab, 2829-511 Caparica, Portugal; mariaalziracavacas6@gmail.com (M.A.C.); pmascarenhas@egasmoniz.edu.pt (P.M.); pedromaoliveira@hotmail.com (P.O.); czagalo1@sapo.pt (C.Z.)
2. Instituto de Anatomia, Faculty of Medicine, University of Lisbon, 1649-028 Lisbon, Portugal
* Correspondence: raquelpacheco77@gmail.com; Tel.: +351-912-470-328
† Presented at the 5th International Congress of CiiEM—Reducing inequalities in Health and Society, Online, 16–18 June 2021.

Abstract: This systematic review and meta-analysis aimed to assess the literature about the incidence of oral mucositis and its degrees (mild, moderate, and severe), in patients undergoing head and neck cancer treatment (radiotherapy, chemotherapy, and surgery). Addressing this issue is important since oral mucositis has a negative impact on oral health and significantly deteriorates the quality of life. Therefore, a multidisciplinary team, including dentists, should be involved in the treatment. The overall oral mucositis incidence was 89.4%. The global incidence for mild, moderate, and severe degrees were 16.8%, 34.5%, and 26.4%, respectively. The high incidence rates reported in this review point out the need for greater care in terms of the oral health of these patients.

Keywords: head and neck cancer; oral mucositis; radiotherapy; chemotherapy

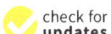

1. Introduction

OM (oral mucositis) is an acute response which affects patients undergoing radiotherapy (RT) and/or chemotherapy (QT) treatments for head and neck cancer. OM includes clinically erosive and/or ulcerative oral lesions that can cause mild to severe pain [1–6]. Due to the overall impact on oral health, it is important to evaluate these patients before and after treatment and to have an effective collaboration between health professionals [4].

2. Materials and Methods

This systematic review assessed the following research question: 'What is the incidence of OM, as well as the respective degrees, in the context of treatment (RT/QT/surgery) of patients with head and neck cancer?' Articles published between 2015 and 2020, adult patients (≥18 years), and articles that present the incidence of OM in patients during and/or after treatment for head and neck cancer were included. The search was carried out using three databases: PubMed, B-on, and Google Scholar. Six articles were included in the systematic review and in the meta-analysis. The formula [OM incidence = patients with OM/total sample] was used to determine the incidence. Random effect meta-analysis statistics and graphs were performed using Open Meta [Analyst] in its current version.

3. Results and Discussion

The studies in this review reported a high incidence of OM (89.4%), as seen in Figure 1. Heterogeneity was close to 81%. Most reported cases of OM were moderate. Partial incidence of degrees 1, 2, and 3 of OM was 16.8%, 34.5%, and 26.4%, respectively.

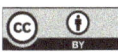

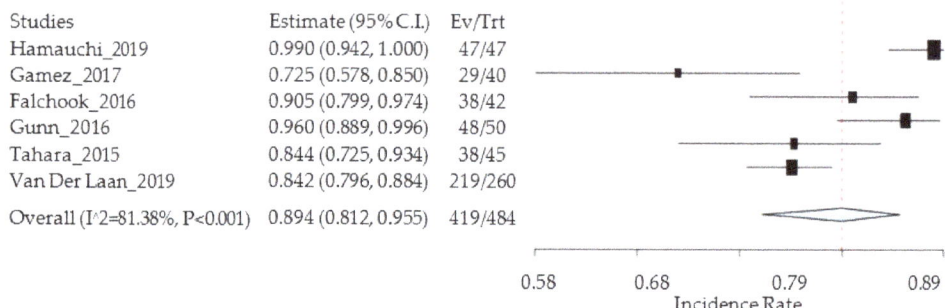

Figure 1. Forest plot representative of the meta-analysis of the incidence rate of OM: Ev—number of patients who had OM and Trt—number of patients who underwent treatment for head and neck cancer at risk of developing OM.

The incidence rates of OM reported in this meta-analysis are high, with a need for greater care in terms of the oral health of these patients. In short, there were some limitations in this systematic review in terms of the number of articles published in the last 5 years in relation to OM. Another major limitation was the great heterogeneity in the treatments that patients were subjected to in the different articles and often within the article itself.

Conflicts of Interest: The authors declare no conflict of interest.

References

1. Hamauchi, S.; Yokota, T.; Mizumachi, T.; Onozawa, Y.; Ogawa, H.; Onoe, T.; Kamijo, T.; Iida, Y.; Nishimura, T.; Onitsuka, T.; et al. Safety and efficacy of concurrent carboplatin or cetuximab plus radiotherapy for locally advanced head and neck cancer patients ineligible for treatment with cisplatin. *Int. J. Clin. Oncol.* **2019**, *24*, 468–475. [CrossRef] [PubMed]
2. Gamez, M.E.; Halyard, M.Y.; Hinni, M.L.; Hayden, R.E.; Nagel, T.H.; Vargas, C.E.; Wong, W.W.; Curtis, K.K.; Zarka, M.A.; Ma, D.; et al. Mucosal Sparing Radiation Therapy in Resected Oropharyngeal Cancer. *Ann. Otol. Rhinol. Laryngol.* **2017**, *126*, 185–191. [CrossRef] [PubMed]
3. Falchook, A.D.; Green, R.; Knowles, M.E.; Amdur, R.J.; Mendenhall, W.; Hayes, D.N.; Grilley-Olson, J.E.; Weiss, J.; Reeve, B.B.; Mitchell, S.A.; et al. Comparison of patient- and practitioner-reported toxic effects associated with chemoradiotherapy for head and neck cancer. *JAMA Otolaryngol. Head Neck Surg.* **2016**, *142*, 517–523. [CrossRef] [PubMed]
4. Gunn, G.B.; Blanchard, P.; Garden, A.S.; Zhu, X.R.; Fuller, C.D.; Mohamed, A.S.; Morrison, W.H.; Phan, J.; Beadle, B.M.; Skinner, H.D.; et al. Clinical Outcomes and Patterns of Disease Recurrence after Intensity Modulated Proton Therapy for Oropharyngeal Squamous Carcinoma. *Int. J. Radiat. Oncol. Biol. Phys.* **2016**, *95*, 360–367. [CrossRef] [PubMed]
5. Tahara, M.; Kiyota, N.; Mizusawa, J.; Nakamura, K.; Hayashi, R.; Akimoto, T.; Hasegawa, Y.; Iwae, S.; Monden, N.; Matsuura, K.; et al. Phase II trial of chemoradiotherapy with S-1 plus cisplatin for unresectable locally advanced head and neck cancer (JCOG0706). *Cancer Sci.* **2015**, *106*, 726–733. [CrossRef] [PubMed]
6. Van Der Laan, B.F.A.M.; Van Der Laan, H.P.; Bijl, H.P.; Steenbakkers, R.J.H.M.; Van Der Schaaf, A.; Chouvalova, O.; Vemer-Van Den Hoek, J.G.M.; Gawryszuk, A.; Oosting, S.F.; Roodenburg, J.L.N.; et al. Acute symptoms during the course of head and neck radiotherapy or chemoradiation are strong predictors of late dysphagia. *Radiat. Oncol.* **2015**, *115*, 56–62. [CrossRef]

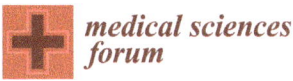

Proceedings

Children's Oral Health on Pico Island, Azores (Portugal) [†]

Juliana Pereira [1,*], Gunel Kizi [2], Ana Raquel Barata [2] and Irene Ventura [2]

1. Egas Moniz Cooperativa de Ensino Superior, C.R.L., 2829-511 Almada, Portugal
2. Centro de investigação interdisciplinar Egas Moniz (CiiEM), Egas Moniz Cooperativa de Ensino Superior, C.R.L., 2829-511 Almada, Portugal; gunelkizi@outlook.com (G.K.); raquelgarciabarata@gmail.com (A.R.B.); imvcr.ireneventura@gmail.com (I.V.)
* Correspondence: julianaapereira1997@gmail.com; Tel.: +351-913320249
† Presented at the 5th International Congress of CiiEM—Reducing inequalities in Health and Society, Online, 16–18 June 2021.

Abstract: Pediatric dentistry focuses on children's oral health. The aim of this study was to describe the prevalence of malocclusion in a pediatric population. Eighty-two children (3–12 years old), of both genders, who belong to a Social Solidarity Institution for Children in Pico Island were clinically examined. Half were female and half were male, in which most were 7 years old (20.7%) with mixed dentition (58.5%). The highest prevalence was in canine class I and vertical molar. Most children did not have malocclusion characteristics (56.1%).

Keywords: prevalence; malocclusion; children

1. Introduction

Pediatric Dentistry focuses on preserving children's oral health, and on preventing and treating diseases of the stomatognathic system observed during childhood and adolescence, from the eruption of the first deciduous tooth to the establishment of permanent occlusion [1]. Malocclusion is one of the most prevalent pathologies in this period, affecting not only the masticatory function but also the cranial development, facial appearance, and the quality of life of affected children. That is why it is so important that dentists must pay attention to the main risk factors and detect the first signs of this condition to intervene as early as possible [2–4]. The aim of this study was to describe the prevalence of malocclusion relating to the age group, gender, and type of dentition of the population sampled.

2. Materials and Methods

An epidemiological and descriptive study was carried out with a sample composed of 82 children, aged between three and twelve years old, of both genders (50% male; 50% female), who belong to a Social Solidarity Institution for Children in Pico Island, Azores (Portugal). The study was approved by the ethics committee of Egas Moniz Higher Education Cooperative, process no 811 of 19 December 2019. Inclusion criteria were children aged between three and twelve years old without craniofacial changes, and children who agreed to participate in the study through the presence of informed consent duly signed by a guardian or other legally responsible adult. Exclusion criteria were children with craniofacial disorders who had already undergone orthodontic treatment, and children who did not accept participation in the study or were not able to provide informed consent. Data were analyzed using descriptive and inferential methodologies. A significance level of 5% was set in the latter case.

3. Results and Discussion

The sample had total homogeneous distribution regarding gender, with 50% of the children female and 50% male, in which most were 7 years old (20.7%) and had mixed dentition (58.5%). Highest prevalence was registered in canine relationship class I, both on the right (79.3%) and on the left (78%). The vertical step also registered the highest prevalence, both on the right (46.3%) and on the left (43.9%). No association was identified between variable malocclusion and the remaining variables. Finally, most children did not have malocclusion characteristics (56.1%) (Table 1). The higher prevalence was registered in canine relationship class I and vertical molar relationship. Most children did not have malocclusion characteristics. It is important to carry out more epidemiological studies in the Azores to understand the panorama of children's oral health and to monitor the evolution of data collected in the target population region of this study.

Table 1. Malocclusion prevalence.

	Frequency	Percentage (%)
Yes	36	43.9
No	46	51.6
Total	82	100

Institutional Review Board Statement: The study was conducted according to the guidelines of the Declaration of Helsinki, and approved by the Ethics Committee of Egas Moniz Higher Education Cooperative, process no 811 of 19 December 2019.

Informed Consent Statement: Informed consent was obtained from all subjects involved in the study. Written informed consent has been obtained from the patient(s) to publish this paper.

Data Availability Statement: MDPI Research Data Policies.

Acknowledgments: Nothing to declare.

Conflicts of Interest: The authors declare no conflict of interest.

References

1. Zou, J.; Meng, M.; Law, C.S.; Rao, Y.; Zhou, X. Common dental diseases in children and malocclusion. *Int. J. Oral Sci.* **2018**, *10*, 7. [CrossRef] [PubMed]
2. Mutlu, E.; Parlak, B.; Kuru, S.; Oztas, E.; Pinar-Erdem, A.; Elif, E. Evaluation of crossbites in relation with dental arch widths, occlusion type, nutritive and non-nutritive sucking habits and respiratory factors in the early mixed dentition. *Oral Health Prev. Dent.* **2019**, *17*, 447–455. [CrossRef] [PubMed]
3. Belfer, M. The Association between the Type of Bad Oral Habit and the Kind of Malocclusion in Children. *SAODS* **2019**, *2*, 24–26.
4. Yu, X.; Zhang, H.; Sun, L.; Pan, J.; Liu, Y.; Chen, L. Prevalence of malocclusion and occlusal traits in the early mixed dentition in Shanghai, China. *PeerJ* **2019**, *7*, e6630. [CrossRef]

Proceeding Paper

Oral Complications of Chemotherapy on Paediatric Patients with Cancer: A Systematic Review and Meta-Analysis †

Ana Sofia Alves [1,*], Gunel Kizi [2], Ana Raquel Barata [2], Paulo Mascarenhas [2] and Irene Ventura [2]

1. Egas Moniz Cooperativa de Ensino Superior, C.R.L., 2829-511 Almada, Portugal
2. Paediatric Dentistry, CiiEM Centro de Investigação Interdisciplinar Egas Moniz, 2829-511 Almada, Portugal; gunelkizi@outlook.com (G.K.); raquelgarciabarata@gmail.com (A.R.B.); pmascarenhas@egasmoniz.edu.pt (P.M.); imvcr.ireneventura@gmail.com (I.V.)
* Correspondence: anasofia.ralves@gmail.com
† Presented at the 5th International Congress of CiiEM—Reducing Inequalities in Health and Society, Online, 16–18 June 2021.

Abstract: The goal of cancer treatment is to fight and/or control cancer. The aim of this study was to review and meta-analyse the incidence of main oral complications in paediatric oncology during chemotherapy. The search results were obtained from B-on, Web of Science, Scopus, Cochrane Library and PubMed databases. Of 1032 articles potentially relevant, 13 were included in this review. The overall incidence of caries, gingivitis, ulcers, mucositis, and candidiasis was 67.8%, 55.6%, 44.2%, 41.6%, and, 29.5%, respectively. During chemotherapy, paediatric patients with cancer present higher incidence of caries and gingivitis. Incidence rate meta-analysis show high heterogeneity. More studies should be done to reduce uncertainty.

Keywords: chemotherapy; paediatric dentistry; oral manifestations

1. Introduction

The goal of cancer treatment is to fight and/or control cancer. Unfortunately, there are no fully selective therapies yet and the body ends up suffering adverse effects that can compromise the patient's quality of life. These therapies and the cancer disease itself are deeply linked to oral health [1–3]. Existing evidence indicates that the chemotherapy used to treat paediatric cancer is associated with disturbances in tooth development, poorer oral hygiene, oral lesions, hyposalivation and an increased prevalence of dental caries when compared to healthy children [4]. The purpose of this systematic review was to assess and summarize impact of disease/treatment interaction on the incidence ratio of caries, gingivitis, ulcers, mucositis and candidiasis. The focused question addressed was: "What are the major oral complications in paediatric patients during chemotherapy?". This study systematically investigates oral complications resulting from chemotherapy treatments in children within a maximum period of 2 years after treatment.

2. Materials and Methods

The search results were obtained from B-on, Web of Science, Scopus, Cochrane Library and PubMed databases. Articles that met the inclusion and exclusion criteria were selected. The inclusion criteria included: (i) studies including cancer patients diagnosed between the ages of 3 and 18; (ii) participants who did not receive cancer treatment during the data collection period; (iii) patients who experienced oral complications after finishing the cancer treatment and the exclusion criteria were: participants who continue cancer treatment or who have finished treatment for more than 2 years. Incidence rates calculation and subsequent meta-analytical plots were performed using OpenMeta [Analyst] and JASP (Version 0.13.1). Heterogeneity was considered high when $I^2 > 50\%$. Subgroup meta-analysis and meta-regressions were used to assess possible effects of factors (geographic region) and covariates (age, latitude [5] and DMFT–caries only), on oral complications incidence.

3. Results and Discussion

Of 1032 articles potentially relevant, 13 were included in this review. The overall incidence of caries, gingivitis, ulcers, mucositis, and candidiasis was 67.8%, 55.6%, 44.2%, 41.6%, and, 29.5%, respectively (Table 1). Meta-regressions of the incidence of caries, ulcers and candidiasis showed positive effects of age ($p < 0.001$). The results of the cumulative meta-analysis suggest a recent increase in the incidence of ulcers and a decrease in the incidence of caries, gingivitis, and mucositis, over the study period. Subgroup meta-analysis indicated that there are significant regional incidence differences among continents (Z Test, $p < 0.05$), only in ulcers and candidiasis this difference was not significant. We believe that these discrepancies may eventually be associated with government measures to prevent caries disease.

Table 1. Meta-analysis incidence rate and heterogeneity levels (% of total).

Meta-Analysis	Incidence Rate	Heterogeneity ($I^2 > 50\%$)
Caries	67.8%	97.06%
Gingivitis	55.6%	98.82%
Ulcers	44.2%	98.12%
Mucositis	41.6%	96.67%
Candidiasis	29.5%	98.24%

During chemotherapy, paediatric patients with cancer present higher incidence of caries and gingivitis (the two more frequent complications). Incidence rate meta-analysis show high heterogeneity. More studies should be done to reduce uncertainty. We believe that the results obtained may be improved if more dental check-ups are performed in order to prevent or, if necessary, treat early, any oral manifestations resulting from chemotherapy treatments. Children's oral hygiene can always be improved with regular visits to the Dentist and with better education/sensitivity by health professionals and family members.

Conflicts of Interest: The authors declare no conflict of interest.

References

1. Peres, P.; De Queiroz, A.M.; Moreira, M.R.; da Silva Faquim, J.P.; Ferrari, M.A.C.M. Odontopediatria Aplicada Ao Câncer Infantil-Manifestações Clínicas e Protocolos de Atendimento. *J. Manag. Prim. Health Care* **2013**, *4*, 191–199. [CrossRef]
2. Parahym, A.M.R.D.C.; Melo, L.R.B.; Morais, V.L.L.; Neves, R.P. Candidiasis in pediatric patients with cancer interned in a university hospital. *Braz. J. Microbiol.* **2009**, *40*, 321. [CrossRef]
3. Ribeiro, I.; de Andrade Lima Neto, E.; Valenca, A.M. Chemotherapy in Pediatric Oncology Patients and the Occurrence of Oral Mucositis. *Int. J. Clin. Pediatr. Dent.* **2019**, *12*, 261–267. [CrossRef]
4. Busenhart, D.M.; Erb, J.; Rigakos, G.; Eliades, T.; Papageorgiou, S.N. Adverse effects of chemotherapy on the teeth and surrounding tissues of children with cancer: A systematic review with meta-analysis. *Oral Oncol.* **2018**, *83*, 64–72. [CrossRef] [PubMed]
5. Latitude and Longitude Finder on Map Get Coordinates. Available online: https://www.latlong.net/ (accessed on 15 June 2020).

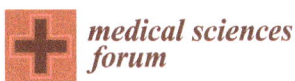

Proceeding Paper

COVID-19 Risk Perception and Confidence among Clinical Dental Students: Impact on Patient Management [†]

Mariana Morgado [1], José João Mendes [1,2] and Luís Proença [2,3,*]

1. Clinical Research Unit (CRU), Centro de Investigação Interdisciplinar Egas Moniz (CiiEM), Egas Moniz—Cooperativa de Ensino Superior CRL, 2829-511 Almada, Portugal; mmorgado@egasmoniz.edu.pt (M.M.); jmendes@egasmoniz.edu.pt (J.J.M.)
2. Evidence-Based Hub, CiiEM, Egas Moniz—Cooperativa de Ensino Superior CRL, 2829-511 Almada, Portugal
3. Quantitative Methods for Health Research (MQIS), CiiEM, Egas Moniz—Cooperativa de Ensino Superior, CRL, 2829-511 Almada, Portugal
* Correspondence: lproenca@egasmoniz.edu.pt
† Presented at the 5th International Congress of CiiEM—Reducing inequalities in Health and Society, Online, 16–18 June 2021.

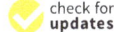

Abstract: This study aimed to assess COVID-19 perceived risk, confidence and its impact on potentially infected patients' management practices, in a clinical dental education setting. The survey was conducted by application of a self-administered questionnaire amid the COVID-19 pandemic. Results indicate high COVID-19 perceived risk and confidence levels (86.7% and 72.8%, respectively). A significantly lower risk perception was identified for individuals classifying COVID-19 as a moderately dangerous disease and confidence was significantly lower for women and for individuals not previously exposed to confirmed or suspected cases of COVID-19. No factor-related significant differences were found on potentially infected patients' management practices.

Keywords: dental education; clinical education; patient management; COVID-19 risk perception

Citation: Morgado, M.; Mendes, J.J.; Proença, L. COVID-19 Risk Perception and Confidence among Clinical Dental Students: Impact on Patient Management. *Med. Sci. Forum* **2021**, *5*, 26. https://doi.org/10.3390/msf2021005026

Academic Editors: Helena Barroso and Cidália Castro

Published: 21 July 2021

Publisher's Note: MDPI stays neutral with regard to jurisdictional claims in published maps and institutional affiliations.

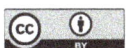

Copyright: © 2021 by the authors. Licensee MDPI, Basel, Switzerland. This article is an open access article distributed under the terms and conditions of the Creative Commons Attribution (CC BY) license (https://creativecommons.org/licenses/by/4.0/).

1. Introduction

COVID-19, caused by the coronavirus SARS-CoV-2, was identified as one of the most impacting infectious diseases of modern times [1]. During the ongoing pandemic period, besides causing a serious threat to human health, COVID-19 had an enormous impact on the education processes, particularly in the clinical context [2]. Due to the inherent characteristics of the clinical dental environment, students face additional challenges, since they have to deal with an emerging infectious disease in the community while conducting their practical learning [3].

A misplaced COVID-19 perceived risk and related confidence can have direct consequences on clinical attitudes and patient management [4].

Thus, it is imperative to study the COVID-19 perceived risk and confidence of dental students, in a clinical context, in order to identify weaknesses in the related health education processes and to find pathways to develop and implement new educational models to use under these circumstances.

2. Materials and Methods

The study included 244 participants, 177 senior under-graduate students and 67 recent graduates from the Integrated Master's Degree in Dentistry conducting their practical learning at Egas Moniz Dental Clinic, a university dental clinic located in the southern Lisbon area (Almada, Portugal). The survey, conducted through the application of an anonymous self-administered questionnaire (SAQ), preceded by informed consent, took place from November 2020 to March 2021, during the most impacting phase of the COVID-19 pandemic in Portugal. COVID-19 self-perceived risk and confidence levels were assessed through numerical scores obtained from the individual answers, expressed in a 5-point Likert scale, to representative questions of each domain. The SAQ was adapted from [1], and its reliability, evaluated using the Cronbach alpha, was 0.64. For ease of data handling and interpretation, the score was converted to a percentage scale. Data were analyzed using descriptive and inferential statistical methodologies. The present work is part of an ongoing research project (Healthcare Education and Pedagogical Innovation) approved by the Egas Moniz Ethics Committee.

3. Results and Discussion

Results indicate an overall high COVID-19 perceived risk and confidence (mean values 86.7% and 72.8%, respectively). No significant differences were found in risk perception when considering a previous infection ($p = 0.499$) or a possible exposition to confirmed or suspected cases ($p = 0.727$). However, a significantly lower risk perception ($p = 0.014$) was identified for individuals classifying COVID-19 as a moderately dangerous disease when comparing with the ones that classify it as very dangerous (mean values 84.4 vs. 87.9%). Confidence was found to be significantly lower for women ($p = 0.001$) and for individuals not previously exposed to confirmed or suspected cases of COVID-19 ($p = 0.027$). No relevant correlation was found between COVID-19 risk perception and confidence levels (rho = 0.07, $p = 0.296$).

When considering the attitudes towards the management of a patient exhibiting SARS-CoV-2 infection-like symptoms, 65.6% reported proceeding with the treatment and asking the patient to go to the hospital afterwards, 26.6% referencing the patient to the hospital without providing treatment and 7.8% refusing to provide dental treatment. Even so, no significant differences were found when accounting for the attitudes and practices in the management of patients exhibiting SARS-CoV-2 infection-like symptoms, as a function of the disease perceived risk ($p = 0.064$) and reported confidence ($p = 0.713$) levels.

In light of these results, it is recommended to improve COVID-19 risk perception and confidence levels by using dedicated measures in the clinical dental education context. This could be achieved by developing more resilient and dedicated clinical educational models, applicable in the context of a global public health emergency, optimizing the public health education of future professionals.

Institutional Review Board Statement: The study was conducted according to the guidelines of the Declaration of Helsinki, and approved by the Ethics Committee of Instituto Universitário Egas Moniz (no. 906 of 26 November 2020).

Informed Consent Statement: Informed consent was obtained from all subjects involved in the study.

Data Availability Statement: The data used to support the findings of this study are available from the corresponding author (L.P.) upon request.

Conflicts of Interest: The authors declare no conflict of interest.

References

1. Ding, Y.; Du, X.; Li, Q.; Zhang, M.; Zhang, Q.; Tan, X.; Liu, Q. Risk perception of coronavirus disease 2019 (COVID-19) and its related factors among college students in China during quarantine. *PLoS ONE* **2020**, *15*, e0237626. [CrossRef] [PubMed]
2. Taghrir, M.H.; Borazjani, R.; Shiraly, R. COVID-19 and Iranian Medical Students; A Survey on Their Related-Knowledge, Preventive Behaviors and Risk Perception. *Arch. Iran Med.* **2020**, *23*, 249–254. [CrossRef] [PubMed]
3. Meng, L.; Hua, F.; Bian, Z. Coronavirus Disease 2019 (COVID-19): Emerging and Future Challenges for Dental and Oral Medicine. *J. Dent. Res.* **2020**, *99*, 481–487. [CrossRef] [PubMed]
4. Almulhim, B.; Alassaf, A.; Alghamdi, S.; Alroomy, R.; Aldhuwayhi, S.; Aljabr, A.; Mallineni, S.K. Dentistry Amidst the COVID-19 Pandemic: Knowledge, Attitude, and Practices Among the Saudi Arabian Dental Students. *Front. Med.* **2021**, *8*, 400. [CrossRef] [PubMed]

Proceeding Paper

Awareness and Use of Heat-Not-Burn Tobacco among Students of Egas Moniz—Cooperative of Higher Education [†]

Ana Sofia Pintado [1,*], Duarte Sousa-Tavares [2] and Patrícia Cavaco-Silva [2]

1. Pharmaceutical Sciences, Egas Moniz University Institute (IUEM), 2829-511 Monte de Caparica, Portugal
2. Egas Moniz Interdisciplinary Center (CiiEM), 2829-511 Monte de Caparica, Portugal; dptavares@egasmoniz.edu.pt (D.S.-T.); montezpat@gmail.com (P.C.-S.)
* Correspondence: sofia.pintado2@gmail.com
† Presented at the 5th International Congress of CiiEM—Reducing inequalities in Health and Society, Online, 16–18 June 2021.

Abstract: Heated tobacco products (HTP) use a device that heats tobacco to generate an aerosol containing nicotine instead of burning it as it happens with combustion tobacco. This study aimed to determine the prevalence of heat-not-burn tobacco use among students of a Healthcare University Institution—Egas Moniz—and identify the factors that influence this use. A questionnaire adapted from the WHO Global Health Professional Students Survey was applied between May and July 2019 in the study population. Subsequently, an exploratory analysis of the data was carried out and a logistic regression was applied in order to determine the factors that influence students to consume heated tobacco.

Keywords: heat-not-burn tobacco; prevalence; college students

1. Introduction

Heated tobacco products (HTP) use a device that heats tobacco to generate an aerosol containing nicotine instead of burning it at significantly higher temperatures, as it happens with combustion tobacco (CT) [1]. This concept was introduced in 1988, however, only in recent years there was an exponential increase in public interest with the launch of the latest HTP in the market [2,3]. Health professionals play a key role in the fight against the tobacco epidemic [4]. The main relevance of this study lies in the fact that there are still no studies on the prevalence of HTP use among college students, in particular, healthcare students.

2. Materials and Methods

An exploratory cross-sectional analytical observational study was carried out. A questionnaire adapted from the WHO Global Health Professional Students Survey (GHPSS) was applied in person between May and July 2019 to the study population, meaning all 3rd year students enrolled at Egas Moniz—a Cooperative of Higher Education dedicated to health sciences—in the academic year 2018–2019 ($n = 389$) [5]. The main variables assessed by the questionnaire were tobacco use prevalence and the factors that influence students to consume heat-not-burn tobacco. Subsequently, an exploratory analysis of the data was carried out providing descriptive information, and a logistic regression was applied in order to determine the factors that influence students to consume heated tobacco. This study was submitted to, and approved by, the Egas Moniz Ethics Commission.

3. Results and Discussion

This study, which covered a sample of 314 participants, demonstrated that 19.93% ($n = 58$) of the students were smokers, 6.87% ($n = 20$) smoked heat-not-burn tobacco and 13.06% ($n = 38$) smoked combustion tobacco (Figure 1), thus, the prevalence of HTP represents more than a third of all smokers (34.47%). This prevalence, 6.8%, is much higher than the prevalence of 0.5% reported recently by Gallus et al., relative to a study conducted in Portugal in 2017 [6].

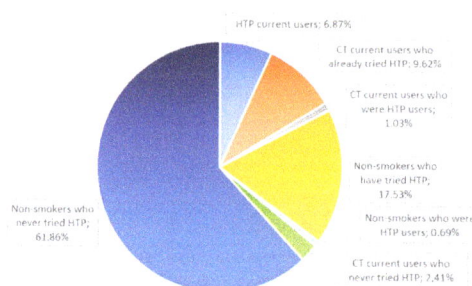

Figure 1. Prevalence of heated tobacco products use and combustion tobacco use among 3rd year students of Egas Moniz—Cooperative of Higher Education, CRL (2019).

Factors That Influence Students to Consume Heat-Not-Burn Tobacco

The students most likely to smoke HTP were the oldest (p-value = 0.070), who considered that HTP should not be banned in indoor public places (p-value < 0.001), who did not know if heated tobacco is more or less harmful compared to conventional cigarettes (p-value = 0.030), and who did not know (p-value = 0.049) or disagreed (p-value = 0.073) that switching from combustion tobacco to a HTP is an approach to smoking cessation.

This study found that about 1/5 of health professional students smoked, of which more than a third were heated tobacco users, which shows that HTP consumption is rising and presents a current public health problem in the health professional university population. As these students are the future health workforce that will provide smoking cessation support, it is important to implement not only tobacco control measures in universities, but also to reinforce academic skills in this area.

Institutional Review Board Statement: The study was conducted according to the guidelines of the Declaration of Helsinki, and approved by the Ethics Committee of Egas Moniz (protocol code nº 756 approved on 2 April 2019).

Informed Consent Statement: Informed consent was obtained from all subjects involved in the study.

Acknowledgments: The authors greatly thank the support of the Egas Moniz Management and teachers, and last but not least, the students, without which this study would have been impossible.

Conflicts of Interest: The authors declare no conflict of interest.

References

1. Ratajczak, A.; Jankowski, P.; Strus, P.; Feleszko, W. Heat Not Burn Tobacco Product—A New Global Trend: Impact of Heat-Not-Burn Tobacco Products on Public Health, a Systematic Review. *Int. J. Environ. Res. Public Health* **2020**, *17*, 409. [CrossRef]
2. Sutherland, G.; Russell, M.; Stapleton, J.; Feyerabend, C. Glycerol particle cigarettes: A less harmful option for chronic smokers. *Thorax* **1993**, *48*, 385–387. [CrossRef]
3. Pokhrel, P.; Herzog, T.A.; Kawamoto, C.T.; Fagan, P. Heat-not-burn Tobacco Products and the Increased Risk for Poly-tobacco Use. *Am. J. Health Behav.* **2021**, *45*, 195–204. [CrossRef]
4. Grech, J.; Sammut, R.; Buontempo, M.B.; Vassallo, P.; Calleja, N. Brief tobacco cessation interventions: Practices, opinions, and attitudes of healthcare professionals. *Tob. Prev. Cessat.* **2020**, *6*, 1–11. [CrossRef]
5. CDC. *Global Health Professional Students*; CDC: Atlanta, GA, USA, 2008.
6. Gallus, S.; Lugo, A.; Liu, X.; Borroni, E.; Clancy, L.; Gorini, G.; Lopez, M.J.; Odone, A.; Przewozniak, K.; Tigova, O.; et al. Use and awareness of heated tobacco products in europe. *J. Epidemiol.* **2021**. [CrossRef]

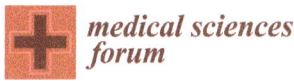

Proceeding Paper

Inflammatory Bowel Disease, Alpha-Synuclein Aggregates and Parkinson's Disease: The InflamaSPark Protocol [†]

Miguel Grunho [1,2,*], Catarina Godinho [1], Marta Patita [3], Irina Mocanu [3], Ana Isabel Vieira [3], António Alves de Matos [4], Ricardo Carregosa [1], Frederico Marx [1], Morgane Tomé [1], Diogo Sousa-Catita [1], Luís Proença [1], Tiago Outeiro [5] and Jorge Fonseca [1,3,*]

1. PaMNEC—Grupo de Patologia Médica, Nutrição e Exercício Clínico/CiiEM—Centro de Investigação Interdisciplinar Egas Moniz, 2829-511 Almada, Portugal; cgodinho@egasmoniz.edu.pt (C.G.); carregosa1978@gmail.com (R.C.); fredmarx1999@gmail.com (F.M.); morgane.ac99@gmail.com (M.T.); diogo.rsc2@gmail.com (D.S.-C.); lproenca@egasmoniz.edu.pt (L.P.)
2. Movement Disorders Outpatient Clinic, Department of Neurology, Hospital Garcia de Orta, 2801-951 Almada, Portugal
3. Gastroenterology Department, Hospital Garcia de Orta, 2801-951 Almada, Portugal; martapatita21@gmail.com (M.P.); irina.mocanu.24@gmail.com (I.M.); anaircvieira@hotmail.com (A.I.V.)
4. Centro de Microscopia Eletrónica e Histopatologia Egas Moniz (Cmicros), 2829-511 Almada, Portugal; apamatos@gmail.com
5. Department of Experimental Neurodegeneration, University Medical Center Göttingen, 37075 Göttingen, Germany; touteiro@gmail.com
* Correspondence: miguelgrunho@gmail.com (M.G.); jorgedafonseca@hotmail.com (J.F.)
† Presented at the 5th International Congress of CiiEM—Reducing Inequalities in Health and Society, Online, 16–18 June 2021.

Abstract: The hallmark of Parkinson's disease (PD) is the accumulation of alpha-synuclein (AS) aggregates. Prior to the central nervous system involvement, PD establishes itself in the gut as a result of the complex interplay between microbiota, the host's immune/neural systems and increased intestinal permeability. Inflammatory Bowel Disease (IBD) patients present a higher number of AS aggregates in the intestinal wall and an increased risk of developing PD. By studying AS aggregates in gut biopsy specimens of IBD patients and controls, this project aims to further clarify the pathophysiology of PD and to explore the potential of gut a biopsy for AS aggregates as a biomarker for prodromal PD.

Keywords: inflammatory bowel disease; gut alpha-synuclein aggregates; Parkinson's disease

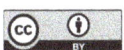

1. Introduction

Recent pathophysiological models of Parkinson's disease (PD) suggest that, prior to the central nervous system involvement, the disease establishes itself peripherally, most likely in the gut, as a result of a complex interplay between the microbiota and the host's immune and neural systems facilitated by changes in intestinal permeability [1]. Inflammatory bowel disease (IBD) is a paradigm of inflammation and disruption of intestinal wall integrity, and provides a favorable setting for the formation of alpha-synuclein (AS) aggregates that characterize PD early stages. IBD patients present a higher number of AS aggregates in the intestinal wall and an increased risk of developing PD (risk ratio of 1.28 for Crohn's disease [CD] and 1.30 for Ulcerative Colitis [UC]) [1]. This study aims to evaluate and characterize the presence of AS aggregates in IBD intestinal biopsies, correlating this presence with clinical features to further clarify the pathophysiological of the PD cascade, and to explore the usefulness of gut AS aggregates as biomarkers for PD diagnosis in prodromal stages. This may prove to be particularly useful for populations at higher risk of PD, such as IBD patients [2].

2. Materials and Methods

This is an observational, noninterventional, case-control study with an 18 months enrollment of IBD patients. Sample: (50 patients/50 controls). (a) Cases: convenience sample from patients with IBD under active follow-up in the IBD Outpatient Clinic of Gastroenterology Department. Inclusion criteria: willingness to participate; ability to understand, provide informed consent and comply with all the proceedings; adult patients with a confirmed diagnosis of IBD according to the appropriate diagnostic criteria under follow-up by a gastroenterologist specialized in IBD. Exclusion criteria: IBD limited to the rectum; comorbidities and/or abnormalities in the physical exam with the potential to develop an undue risk during the procedures; clinical suspicion or prior diagnosis of synucleinopathy. (b) Controls: convenience sample from consenting patients undergoing upper and/or lower gastrointestinal endoscopy, whose biopsies, obtained from normal-appearing mucosa, are considered exempt from changes of pathological significance. Variables: demographics; general clinical data; screening for motor and nonmotor symptoms of PD; evaluation of olfaction and IBD-related data (just for the cases). (a) IBD clinical data: age at diagnosis, type (CD or UC) and phenotype of IBD, disease activity, history of surgical procedures and admissions related to IBD, as well as the ongoing and previous medication related to IBD. (b) IBD laboratory data: fecal calprotectin and serum c-reactive protein levels. Processing and analysis of gut biopsies. (1) Optical microscopy (OM): standard analysis in clinical practice for structural and histological characterization. (2) Immunohistochemistry: identification/quantification of AS aggregates in the gut wall of patients and controls. (3) Electron microscopy: ultrastructural analysis of the tissue. At this stage, only the samples of the subjects with high burden of AS aggregates on OM will be evaluated (top 10% of cases and top 10% of controls). Appropriate statistical analysis will be performed. The project will be conducted in accordance with the Helsinki Declaration and will seek approval by the local Ethics Committees. Data collection/analysis will be conducted in compliance with all ethical principles, including proper protection of confidentiality of the participants.

3. Results and Discussion

In line with the current knowledge in this field, we expect to find that compared to controls: (1) IBD patients have a higher burden of AS intestinal aggregates, mainly those with more disease activity/poor response to treatment and, as such, more inflammation and disruption of intestinal wall integrity; and (2) IBD patients have more motor and nonmotor clinical markers of prodromal PD. Additionally, by employing electron microcopy techniques, we expect to fully characterize the AS aggregates at an ultrastructural level. Since the research will be conducted on human subjects (not animal models) with a higher theoretical risk of developing PD (IBD patients), from a "real-world" clinical setting, our results can be a valuable contribution to the field. Ultimately, the InflamaSPark has the potential to further elucidate the complex and mostly unknown cascade of events that occurs in the gut at the prodromal stages of PD.

Institutional Review Board Statement: The study was conducted according to the guidelines of the Declaration of Helsinki, and approved by the Institutional Review Board of Instituto Universitário Egas Moniz (protocol code 113/2021; date of approval: 8 July 2021).

Informed Consent Statement: Not applicable.

Data Availability Statement: Not applicable.

Conflicts of Interest: The authors declare no conflict of interest.

References

1. Brudek, T. Inflammatory Bowel Diseases and Parkinson's Disease. *J. Parkinson's Dis.* **2019**, *9*, S331–S344. [CrossRef] [PubMed]
2. Zhu, F.; Li, C.; Gong, J.; Zhu, W.; Gu, L.; Li, N. The risk of Parkinson's disease in inflammatory bowel disease: A systematic review and meta-analysis. *Dig. Liver Dis.* **2019**, *51*, 38–42. [CrossRef] [PubMed]

Proceeding Paper

Nutritional and Motor Functional Status in Parkinson's Disease: The NutriSPark Protocol [†]

Miguel Grunho [1,2,*], Catarina Godinho [1], Diogo Sousa-Catita [1], Filipa Vicente [1], Luís Proença [1], Ricardo Carregosa [1], Frederico Marx [1], Morgane Tomé [1], Josefa Domingos [1,3] and Jorge Fonseca [1,4]

1. PaMNEC—Grupo de Patologia Médica, Nutrição e Exercício Clínico, CiiEM—Centro de Investigação Interdisciplinar Egas Moniz, 2829-511 Almada, Portugal; cgodinho@egasmoniz.edu.pt (C.G.); diogo.rsc2@gmail.com (D.S.-C.); filipavicente@hotmail.com (F.V.); lproenca@egasmoniz.edu.pt (L.P.); carregosa1978@gmail.com (R.C.); fredmarx1999@gmail.com (F.M.); morgane.ac99@gmail.com (M.T.); domingosjosefa@gemial.com (J.D.); jorgedafonseca@hotmail.com (J.F.)
2. Department of Neurology, Hospital Garcia de Orta, 2801-951 Almada, Portugal
3. Health Coordinator of Portuguese Association of Parkinson's Disease Patients (APDPk), 1070-023 Lisboa, Portugal
4. GENE—Artificial Feeding Team, Gastroenterology Department, Hospital Garcia de Orta, 2801-951 Almada, Portugal
* Correspondence: miguelgrunho@gmail.com
† Presented at the 5th International Congress of CiiEM—Reducing inequalities in Health and Society, Online, 16–18 June 2021.

Abstract: A growing body of evidence suggests that nutritional status may play an important role in the development and course of Parkinson's disease (PD). Nutritional status is known to influence PD motor and non-motor features and is in turn influenced by disease duration and severity. A proper nutritional status assessment and intervention should be incorporated in the management and follow-up of PD patients. This study aims to characterize the impact of nutritional status in multiple domains of PD and to explore the feasibility and the effectiveness of a customized and intensive nutritional intervention compared to standard care.

Keywords: Parkinson's disease; nutritional status; motor function

1. Introduction

Gastrointestinal impairment, such as constipation and delayed gastric emptying, are commonly observed at all stages of Parkinson's disease (PD) and are often overlooked and under-reported in patient interviews, especially in the early stages of PD [1]. A growing body of evidence suggests that nutrition and nutritional status may play an important role in PD [2]. There is preliminary data suggesting that some nutrients may increase an individual's risk for PD, while others may be neuroprotective. In PD patients the disease-related risk of malnutrition adds to the frequent age-related one, becoming an important contributor to poor quality of life (QoL) [3]. A proper nutritional status assessment and intervention should be incorporated in the management and follow-up of people with Parkinson's disease (PwP). In order to reduce the gaps in this area, this project pretends to characterize the neurological, nutritional, and functional status in PwP to determine the relationship between nutritional status, disease severity, motor and non-motor features, depression, cognition, and QoL, and to explore the feasibility and effectiveness of a three-month intensive, customized nutritional intervention, the "NutriSPark protocol", compared to standard care.

2. Materials and Methods

This study is a multicenter, prospective, interventional, randomized, single-blinded study with an active enrollment extending for 15 months. The inclusion criteria are adult patients with a confirmed PD diagnosis according to the appropriate clinical criteria followed up by an examination performed by a neurologist specialized in movement disorders and a willingness to participate in the study. The exclusion criteria are PwP unwilling or unable to provide inform consent, unable to fully understand and respond to questionnaires, already following specific diets or taking nutritional supplements, or with other medical conditions likely to cause malnutrition.

Protocol stages: T0—Baseline: demographics; clinical data and PD features; neurological evaluation of PD; evaluation of depression; cognitive assessment; evaluation of QoL; physical assessment; nutritional assessment; anthropometric measurements; laboratory data; and grip strength evaluation via dynamometry. T1—Nutritional Intervention and Follow-up. The type of nutritional intervention and counseling will be optimized for each subject and will last for three months. The initial nutritional appointment will be similar for all subjects, who will then be randomized into two groups: (1) "intensive/customized nutritional intervention"—"NutriSPark protocol"; (2) "standard care". In this study, the nutritional goal is 1.2–1.5 g/Kg/day of protein. The protein intake will consider the schedule of the levodopa-containing medications prescribed by the neurologist. Each month the "NutriSPark protocol" group will have nutritional appointments to optimize the nutritional intervention. Halfway between the nutritional appointments, a phone call will be made to monitor and troubleshoot any problems concerning the nutritional care plan. The "standard care" group will receive a generic (but adapted to the clinical setting) flyer/brochure with nutritional information for PwP. T2—Re-evaluation and End of Intervention Visit: At the end of the three-month nutritional intervention, all subjects will be re-evaluated (assessment similar to the baseline). Except for the researchers directly involved in the nutritional care, the investigators and raters (e.g., neurologist) will be blinded for the type of nutritional care that the subjects received. Appropriate statistical analysis will be performed.

The NutriSPark project will be conducted in accordance with the Helsinki Declaration and will seek approval by the local Ethics Committee. Data collection and analysis will be conducted in compliance with all ethical principles, including proper protection of the confidentiality of the participants.

3. Results and Discussion

In accordance with the current knowledge in this field, we expect PD patients to underperform in both functional and nutritional assessments. In addition, we expect to confirm that poorer functional/nutritional status in PwP correlates with disease severity, motor and non-motor features, depression, cognition, and QoL. Finally, if the three-month intensive and customized nutritional intervention of NutriSPark proves feasible and effective, it might lead to meaningful changes in the clinical management of PD.

Institutional Review Board Statement: The study was conducted according to the guidelines of the Declaration of Helsinki, and approved by the Institutional Review Board of Instituto Universitário Egas Moniz (protocol code 113/2021; date of approval: 8 July 2021).

Informed Consent Statement: Not applicable.

Data Availability Statement: Not applicable.

Conflicts of Interest: The authors declare no conflict of interest.

References

1. Klingelhoefer, L.; Reichmann, H. The Gut and Nonmotor Symptoms in Parkinson's Disease. *Int. Rev. Neurobiol.* **2017**, *134*, 787–809. [CrossRef] [PubMed]
2. Essat, M.; Archer, R.; Williams, I.; Zarotti, N.; Coates, E.; Clowes, M.; Beever, D.; Hackney, G.; White, S.; Stavroulakis, T.; et al. Interventions to promote oral nutritional behaviours in people living with neurodegenerative disorders of the motor system: A systematic review. *Clin. Nutr.* **2020**, *39*, 2547–2556. [CrossRef] [PubMed]
3. Bianchi, V.E.; Herrera, P.F.; Laura, R. Effect of nutrition on neurodegenerative diseases. A systematic review. *Nutr. Neurosci.* **2019**, *2019*, 1–25. [CrossRef] [PubMed]

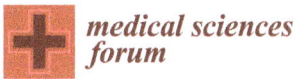

Proceeding Paper

Adverse Childhood Experiences and Empathy: The Role of Interparental Conflict [†]

Ana V. Antunes [1], Patrícia Oliveira [1,*], Jorge Cardoso [1,2] and Telma C. Almeida [1,2]

1. LabPSI–Laboratório de Psicologia Egas Moniz, Instituto Universitário Egas Moniz, 2829-511 Almada, Portugal; ana.vanessa.antunes@gmail.com (A.V.A.); jorgecardoso.psi@gmail.com (J.C.); telma.c.almeida@gmail.com (T.C.A.)
2. CiiEM–Centro de Investigação Interdisciplinar Egas Moniz, Instituto Universitário Egas Moniz (IUEM), Caparica, 2829-511 Almada, Portugal
* Correspondence: patriciasofia_27@hotmail.com
† Presented at the 5th International Congress of CiiEM—Reducing Inequalities in Health and Society, Online, 16–18 June 2021.

Abstract: The literature shows that adverse life experiences may harm individuals. The main objectives of this research were to study the relationship between adverse childhood experiences and empathy in adulthood and analyse differences between victims and nonvictims of interparental conflict. Our research evidenced that adverse childhood experiences affect individuals' empathy in adulthood, and victims of interparental violence experienced other childhood victimization.

Keywords: adverse childhood experiences; empathy; interparental conflict

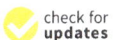

1. Introduction

Adverse childhood experiences (ACE) have a negative impact in the short and long term on victims' lives. Some authors define ACE as the experience of emotional abuse, sexual abuse, physical abuse, emotional neglect and physical neglect, parental divorce, exposure to violence, substance abuse, mental illness or suicide in the family environment, and/or the arrest of a family member [1,2]. The impact of adverse experiences in childhood can be established at psychological, emotional, social, and behavioural levels in adulthood [3]. Some studies reported a relationship between child abuse and the lack of empathy [4]. Empathy is a multidimensional concept that includes affective, cognitive, and behavioural aspects and implies knowing what a person feels [5–7]. The severity of ACE regulates empathy, affecting individuals' relationships [8]. The experience of a disruptive and hostile family environment (e.g., interparental conflict) may result in a lack of empathy, being a facilitator of aggressive and antisocial behaviour in the victim. That may affect the development of individual's empathy showing a history of more unstable and less satisfying intimate relationships [6,8–10].

2. Materials and Methods

This study comprised 119 Portuguese adults (73.1% women and 26.9% men) with ages between 19 and 77 years ($M = 41.91$, $SD = 12.65$), of which 79 (66.4%) were victims of interparental conflict. Participants answered online to the sociodemographic questionnaire, the Adverse Childhood Experiences (ACE), and the Portuguese Interpersonal Reactivity Index (IRI). The ACE assess the degree of exposure to adverse childhood experiences [2], and the IRI assess empathy [5]. Informed consent was obtained, and this study was conducted following the ethical principles outlined in the Declaration of Helsinki [11].

3. Results and Discussion

The results showed statistically significant negative correlations between physical neglect and personal discomfort ($r = -0.18$, $p = 0.47$) and between emotional neglect and

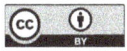

perspective-taking ($r = -0.18$, $p = 0.48$). Household substance abuse ($r = 0.22$, $p = 0.02$) and mental illness or suicide in the family ($r = 0.22$, $p = 0.01$), showed positive correlations with personal discomfort, which corroborates the literature [4]. We also found that participants who were victims of interparental conflict in their childhood had more experiences of emotional ($M = 9.40$, $DP = 17.70$), ($F (1,117) = 6.69$, $p = 0.003$) and physical abuse ($M = 12.15$, $DP = 24.27$), ($F (1,117) = 9.99$, $p = 0.002$), household substance abuse ($M = 18.99$, $DP = 26.92$), ($F (1,117) = 7.47$, $p = 0.007$), and mental illness or suicide in the family ($M = 22.78$, $DP = 32.81$), ($F (1,117) = 7.14$, $p = 0.009$) than nonvictims. These results follow the outcomes of other studies concerning the probability of experiencing several types of victimization [12]. Considering these results, it is crucial to develop preventive programs with children and intervention with individuals who experienced ACE, promoting empathy training [8]. For future studies, we propose to compare individuals with different ages, sex, and levels of resilience, who had suffered childhood ACE to study empathy differences in adulthood.

Institutional Review Board Statement: The study was conducted according to the guidelines of the Declaration of Helsinki.

Informed Consent Statement: Informed consent was obtained from all subjects involved in the study.

Conflicts of Interest: The authors declare no conflict of interest.

References

1. Anda, R.F.; Croft, J.B.; Felitti, V.J.; Nordenberg, D.; Giles, W.H.; Williamson, D.F.; Giovino, G.A. Adverse childhood experiences and smoking during adolescence and adulthood. *Am. Med Assoc.* **1999**, *282*, 1652–1658. [CrossRef] [PubMed]
2. Pinto, R.; Correia, L.; Maia, A. Assessing the reliability of retrospective reports of adverse childhood experiences among adolescents with documented childhood maltreatment. *J. Fam. Violence* **2014**, *29*, 431–438. [CrossRef]
3. Cecconello, A.M.; Koller, S.H. Competência social e empatia: Um estudo sobre resiliência com crianças em situação de pobreza. *Estud. Psicol.* **2000**, *5*, 71–93. [CrossRef]
4. Straker, G.; Jacobson, R.S. Aggression, emotional maladjustment, and empathy in the abused child. *Dev. Psychol.* **1981**, *17*, 762–765. [CrossRef]
5. Limpo, T.; Alves, R.A.; Catro, S.L. Medir a empatia: Adaptação portuguesa do índice de reatividade interpessoal. *Laboratório Psicol.* **2010**, *8*, 171–184. [CrossRef]
6. Parlar, M.; Frewen, P.; Nazarov, A.; Oremus, C.; MacQueen, G.; Lanius, R.; McKinnon, M.C. Alterations in empathic responding among women with posttraumatic stress disorder associated with childhood trauma. *Brain Behav.* **2014**, *4*, 381–389. [CrossRef]
7. Sampaio, L.R.; Camino, C.P.S.; Roazzi, A. Revisão de aspectos conceituais, teóricos e metodológicos da empatia. *Psicol. Ciência e Profissão* **2009**, *29*, 212–227. [CrossRef]
8. Locher, S.C.; Barenblatt, L.; Fourie, M.M.; Stein, D.J.; Gobodo-Madikizela, P. Empathy and childhood maltreatment: A mixed-methods investigation. *Ann. Clin. Psychiatry* **2014**, *26*, 97–110. [PubMed]
9. Godbout, N.; Dutton, D.G.; Lussier, Y.; Sabourin, S. Early exposure to violence, domestic violence, attachment representations, and marital adjustment. *Pers. Relatsh.* **2009**, *16*, 365–384. [CrossRef]
10. Maneta, E.K.; Cohen, S.; Schulz, M.S.; Waldinger, R.J. Linkages between childhood emotional abuse and marital satisfaction: The mediating role of empathic accuracy for hostile emotions. *Child Abus. Negl.* **2015**, *44*, 8–17. [CrossRef] [PubMed]
11. World Medical Association. World medical association declaration of Helsinki: Ethical principles for medical research involving human subjects. *JAMA* **2013**, *310*, 2191–2194. [CrossRef] [PubMed]
12. Almeida, T.C.; Ramos, C.; Brito, J.; Cardoso, J. The Juvenile Victimization Questionnaire: Psychometric properties and polyvictimization among Portuguese youth. *Child. Youth Serv. Rev.* **2013**, *113*. [CrossRef]

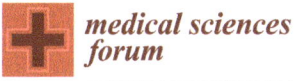

Proceeding Paper

Gut Status in Parkinson's Disease: The GutSPark Protocol [†]

Miguel Grunho [1,2,*], Catarina Godinho [1], António Alves de Matos [3], Helena Barroso [4], Ricardo Carregosa [1], Frederico Marx [1], Morgane Tomé [1], Josefa Domingos [1,5], Diogo Sousa-Catita [1], João Botelho [1], Vanessa Machado [1], José João Mendes [1], Tiago Outeiro [6] and Jorge Fonseca [1,7]

1. PaMNEC—Grupo de Patologia Médica, Nutrição e Exercício Clínico/CiiEM—Centro de Investigação Interdisciplinar Egas Moniz, 2829-511 Almada, Portugal; cgodinho@egasmoniz.edu.pt (C.G.); carregosa1978@gmail.com (R.C.); fredmarx1999@gmail.com (F.M.); morgane.ac99@gmail.com (M.T.); domingosjosefa@gmail.com (J.D.); diogo.rsc2@gmail.com (D.S.-C.); joaobotelho09@gmail.com (J.B.); vanessamachado558@gmail.com (V.M.); jmendes@egasmoniz.edu.pt (J.J.M.); jorgedafonseca@hotmail.com (J.F.)
2. Movement Disorders Outpatient Clinic, Department of Neurology, Hospital Garcia de Orta, 2801-951 Almada, Portugal
3. Centro de Microscopia Eletrónica e Histopatologia Egas Moniz (Cmicros), 2829-511 Almada, Portugal; apamatos@gmail.com
4. Applied Microbiology Lab—Egas Moniz, 2829-511 Almada, Portugal; mhbarroso@egasmoniz.edu.pt
5. Health Coordinator of Portuguese Association of Parkinson's Disease Patients (APDPk), 1070-023 Lisboa, Portugal
6. Department of Experimental Neurodegeneration, University Medical Center Göttingen, 37075 Göttingen, Germany; touteiro@gmail.com
7. GENE—Artificial Feeding Team, Gastroenterology Department, Hospital Garcia de Orta, 2801-951 Almada, Portugal
* Correspondence: miguelgrunho@gmail.com
† Presented at the 5th International Congress of CiiEM—Reducing Inequalities in Health and Society, Online, 16–18 June 2021.

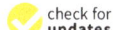

Citation: Grunho, M.; Godinho, C.; de Matos, A.A.; Barroso, H.; Carregosa, R.; Marx, F.; Tomé, M.; Domingos, J.; Sousa-Catita, D.; Botelho, J.; et al. Gut Status in Parkinson's Disease: The GutSPark Protocol. *Med. Sci. Forum* **2021**, *5*, 31. https://doi.org/10.3390/msf2021005031

Academic Editors: Helena Barroso and Cidália Castro

Published: 21 July 2021

Publisher's Note: MDPI stays neutral with regard to jurisdictional claims in published maps and institutional affiliations.

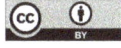

Copyright: © 2021 by the authors. Licensee MDPI, Basel, Switzerland. This article is an open access article distributed under the terms and conditions of the Creative Commons Attribution (CC BY) license (https://creativecommons.org/licenses/by/4.0/).

Abstract: The neuropathological hallmark of Parkinson's disease (PD) is the accumulation of alpha–synuclein (AS) aggregates. The identification of AS aggregates in gut biopsy specimens from people with PD may provide an opportunity to identify PD at a very early stage, prior to symptom onset. Changes in gut microbiota and inflammatory conditions (such as periodontitis) may be linked with PD onset/evolution. This project aims to explore the concept of microbiota–gut–brain axis in PD, studying gut biopsy specimens for AS aggregates, oral and intestinal microbiota, associated digestive disorders and oral health, of both patients with PD and controls.

Keywords: Parkinson's disease; alpha-synuclein; microbiota–gut–brain axis

1. Introduction

The neuropathological hallmark of Parkinson's disease (PD) is the accumulation of misfolded alpha–synuclein (AS) aggregates, leading to neuronal loss in the *substantia nigra* and to dopamine deficiency in the striatum. Both the identification of AS aggregates in gut biopsy specimens from people with PD (PwP) and the reports that this is already evident in prodromal PD open an window of opportunity to identify AS disorders prior to symptoms onset, including PD [1]. Up-to-date pathophysiological models suggest that, prior to central nervous system involvement, the disease establishes peripherally, most likely in the gut, as a result of an intricate interplay between gut microbiota, the host's immune and neural systems, and changes in the intestinal wall permeability—the concept behind the microbiota–gut–brain axis hypothesis [2]. Several studies have explored the connection between PD and certain inflammatory conditions (such as periodontitis) that were found to be interconnected with PD at different disease stages. A shift in gut microbiota, another key component, may facilitate local AS aggregation and the ascending spreading from the enteric nervous system to the brain. The GutSPark study, with its multidisciplinary essence, further explores the concept of the microbiota–gut–brain axis in PD.

The study aims to: (1) To evaluate symptoms of gastrointestinal dysfunction in PwP; (2) To identify and describe oral health problems among PwP; (3) To study the gut, oral and nasal microbiota in PwP; (4) To confirm the presence of, and to characterize, alpha–synuclein aggregates in gut biopsy specimens of patients with PD; (5) To study the microbiome in gut biopsy specimens of patients with PD; (6) To correlate the burden of gastrointestinal dysfunction, oral health problems, microbiota dysbiosis and gut alpha–synuclein aggregates with disease duration, severity, motor and nonmotor features, ongoing treatment, depression and quality of life (QoL) in PwP.

2. Materials and Methods

This is an observational, non-interventional, case-control pilot study, with an enrollment of 18 months. Sample (50 PwP/50 controls): (1) Cases: convenience sample from consenting PwP under active follow-up (Neurology Department of Hospital Garcia de Orta or Portuguese Association of PwP) suitable for enrollment (willingness to participate; ability to understand, provide informed consent and comply with all the proceedings; adult patients with confirmed PD diagnosis according to the appropriate clinical criteria; clinical indication for endoscopy); (2) Controls: convenience sample from consenting patients undergoing upper/lower gastrointestinal endoscopy in the Gastroenterology Department, whose biopsy samples from normal-appearing mucosa are considered exempt from pathological changes. Variables: Demographics; General clinical data; PD-related data (for the cases); Screening for non-motor symptoms of PD; Cognitive screening; Evaluation of QoL; Evaluation of Depression; Digestive symptoms evaluation; and Full-mouth examination. Collection, analysis and processing of the biological samples: samples of oral, nasal swabs, feces and endoscopic biopsies obtained from PwP and controls will be processed in order to characterize the microbiota. Processing and analysis of gut biopsy specimens obtained during endoscopy will be fourfold: (1) Optical microscopy, for histological analysis; (2) Immunohistochemistry, for identification/quantification of gut AS aggregates; (3) Electron microscopy, for ultrastructural analysis; (4) Microbiome study. The project will be conducted in accordance with the Helsinki Declaration and will seek approval by the local Ethics Committee. Data collection and analysis will be conducted in compliance with all ethical principles, including appropriate protection of confidentiality of the participants.

3. Results and Discussion

According to the current knowledge in this field, we expect PD patients to have, comparing to controls, more gastrointestinal dysfunction, oral health problems, microbiota dysbiosis, and alpha–synuclein aggregates in gut biopsy specimens. Furthermore, we expect to confirm a change in the balance of gut/oral/nasal microbiota towards a more proinflammatory milieu in PD. Overall, these changes are expected to correlate with several of the features of PD (disease duration, severity, motor and nonmotor symptoms, ongoing treatment, depression and QoL) and might provide clues to novel treatment targets and/or approaches in this clinical setting.

Institutional Review Board Statement: The study was conducted according to the guidelines of the Declaration of Helsinki, and approved by the Institutional Review Board of Instituto Universitário Egas Moniz (protocol code 113/2021; date of approval: 8 July 2021).

Informed Consent Statement: Not applicable.

Data Availability Statement: Not applicable.

Conflicts of Interest: The authors declare no conflict of interest.

References

1. Klingelhoefer, L.; Reichmann, H. Pathogenesis of Parkinson disease—The gut-brain axis and environmental factors. *Nat. Rev. Neurol.* **2015**, *11*, 625–636. [CrossRef] [PubMed]
2. Lubomski, M.; Tan, A.H.; Lim, S.Y.; Holmes, A.J.; Davis, R.L.; Sue, C.M. Parkinson's disease and the gastrointestinal microbiome. *J. Neurol.* **2020**, *267*, 2507–2523. [CrossRef] [PubMed]

Proceeding Paper

Cow's Milk Protein Allergy: The Hidden Danger of Medicines' Excipients †

Maria Santo, Maria D. Auxtero, Alexandra Figueiredo and Isabel Margarida Costa *

PharmSci Lab-CiiEM, Interdisciplinary Research Center Egas Moniz, Instituto Universitário Egas Moniz, Quinta da Granja, Monte de Caparica, 2829-511 Almada, Portugal; mariahenri@gmail.com (M.S.); mauxtero@egasmoniz.edu.pt (M.D.A.); afigueiredo@egasmoniz.edu.pt (A.F.)

* Correspondence: isabelc@egasmoniz.edu.pt
† Presented at the 5th International Congress of CiiEM—Reducing Inequalities in Health and Society, Online, 16–18 June 2021.

Abstract: In patients with a cow's milk protein allergy, the presence of these allergens in medicines, even in trace amounts, can trigger serious allergic reactions. The study of milk-related excipient prevalence in 165 antiasthmatic medicines, based on the information included in the Summary of Product Characteristics, revealed the presence of lactose in more than one third of these medicines. Since lactose may suffer cross-contamination with cow's milk protein, these results are an alert to health professionals.

Keywords: excipients; lactose; cow's milk protein allergy

1. Introduction

Food allergies are increasingly common, as well as a public health issue with a great impact. Cow's milk protein (CMP) allergy is one of the most common pediatric allergies [1]. CMP allergy may occur at any age. However, it is more prevalent in children under the age of three. In Europe, the reported prevalence ranges from 2% to 7.5% in the first year of life [2]. It is characterized by an immune response to proteins that are present in cow's milk [1]. The symptoms include cutaneous, gastrointestinal and respiratory effects. It is also one of the most common causes of anaphylaxis in children up to 2 years old [3]. Patients with this allergy should exclude milk from their diet [1]. Even dairy products that do not directly contain CMP can trigger an allergic reaction in sensitive patients due to cross-contamination. The intake of medicines containing milk-related excipients, such as lactose, may originate symptoms in allergic patients. This study aimed to evaluate the prevalence of milk derivatives as excipients in antiasthmatic medicines available in Portugal.

2. Materials and Methods

The presence of milk-related excipients was evaluated in 165 antiasthmatic medicines based on the Summary of Product Characteristics (SmPC). Selection criteria of medicines included: marketing authorization approved in Portugal, with the SmPC available on the human medicinal products database (INFOMED), for adult and/or pediatric use, in any dose or dosage form, branded or generic.

3. Results and Discussion

From a total of 165 medicines studied, 99 included lactose as an excipient, as stated in the SmPC, mainly inhalation powders and tablets (Figure 1a). Lactose was the only allergen derived from milk mentioned in the list of excipients. Regarding the presence of the allergen in generic (N = 17) and branded (N = 148) medicines, there is lactose in both groups (Figure 1b), with a similar prevalence (60.1% and 58.8%, respectively).

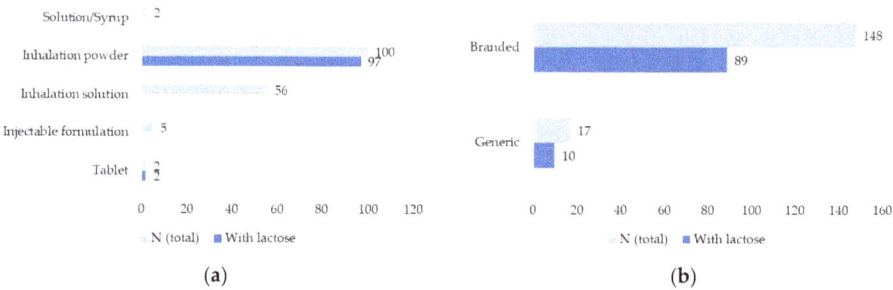

Figure 1. Presence of lactose as excipient according to: (**a**) dosage form; (**b**) generic or branded.

This study revealed a high prevalence of lactose (60%) in antiasthmatic medicines, which may represent a high risk to patients allergic to milk. The presence of milk derivatives as excipients in pharmaceutical products could induce an allergic reaction in patients with CMP allergy. Since respiratory symptoms, such as wheezing, shortness of breath, chest tightness, coughing, and breathing difficulties, are common in allergic patients, antiasthmatics are frequently prescribed medicines.

Lactose, although it is not a milk protein, can also trigger adverse reactions in patients with CMP allergy, due to the risk of cross-contamination by traces of CMP [4]. In the pharmaceutical industry, lactose is widely used as an excipient in medicines [5]. It is used in capsules and tablets as a volume expander or for direct compression, and also as a vehicle in dry powder inhalers, facilitating the delivery of the drug down to the smallest airways [5].

It is essential that the presence of food allergens is highlighted in the composition of the medicines, because even in trace amounts, they can trigger serious reactions in allergic patients. It is also imperative that healthcare professionals have easy access to the detailed composition of medicines, in order to provide a safe prescription and counseling.

Institutional Review Board Statement: Not applicable.

Informed Consent Statement: Not applicable.

Data Availability Statement: Data available in a publicly accessible repository, the data presented in this study are openly available in https://extranet.infarmed.pt/INFOMED-fo/.

Conflicts of Interest: The authors declare no conflict of interest.

References

1. Meng, C.; Sutherland, A.; Birrueta, G.; Laubach, S.; Leonard, S.; Peters, B.; Schulten, V. Analysis of Allergen-Specific T Cell and IgE Reactivity to Different Preparations of Cow's Milk-Containing Food Extracts. *Cells* **2019**, *8*, 667. [CrossRef]
2. European Medicines Agency—Committee for Medicinal Products for Human Use. *Information for the Package Leaflet Regarding Lactose Used as an Excipient in Medicinal Products for Human Use*; European Medicines Agency: London, UK, 2018; EMA/CHMP/186428/2016.
3. Anagnostou, K. Anaphylaxis in Children: Epidemiology, Risk Factors and Management. *Curr. Pediatr. Rev.* **2018**, *14*, 180–186. [CrossRef] [PubMed]
4. Spiegel, W.A.; Anolik, R. Lack of Milk Protein Allergic Reactions in Patients Using Lactose Containing Dry Powder Inhalers (DPIs). *J. Allergy Clin. Immunol.* **2010**, *125*, AB69. [CrossRef]
5. Mill, D.; Dawson, J.; Johnson, J.L. Managing acute pain in patients who report lactose intolerance: The safety of an old excipient re-examined. *Ther. Adv. Drug Saf.* **2018**, *9*, 227–235. [CrossRef] [PubMed]

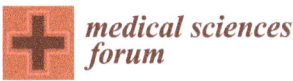

Proceeding Paper

Patient Compliance with Oral Anticoagulant Therapy [†]

Sérgio Valério [1,2,*] and Maria João Hilário [1,2]

1. Higher Education School Egas Moniz, 2829-511 Almada, Portugal; mjhilario1973@gmail.com
2. Lisbon North University Hospital Center, 1649-028 Lisboa, Portugal
* Correspondence: sfcvalerio@gmail.com
† Presented at the 5th International Congress of CiiEM—Reducing Inequalities in Health and Society, Online, 16–18 June 2021.

Abstract: Oral anticoagulants (OAC) are intended to enhance the unwanted activation of blood clotting, and they are used for the prophylaxis and treatment of thromboembolic events. This study aimed to describe and verify whether there was a relationship between patient compliance with OAC therapy and patient gender and age, using a sample of 111 individuals. The data were collected through individual forms, from patients in a Hospital Unit in Great Lisbon. Results showed a statistically significant relationship between patient compliance with OAC therapy and the variables gender and age.

Keywords: oral anticoagulants; compliance; hypocoagulated

1. Introduction

Oral anticoagulants (OACs), as anti-vitamin K drugs, are characterized by preventing the carboxylation of coagulation factors II, VII, IX, and X, leading to the synthesis of inactive factors [1]. They are used in diseases that potentiate an unwanted activation of blood coagulation, used for the prophylaxis and treatment of thromboembolic events [1].

Therapy with OACs consists of the oral administration of the drug. Its dosage varies according to the assessment of the clinician and laboratory analyses (international normalized ratio—INR) [2].

Indications for OAC include the prevention and treatment of venous thromboembolism, pulmonary thromboembolism, acute myocardial infarction, valve prostheses, and atrial fibrillation, among others [3].

Anticoagulation stability is related to patient compliance, as well as several other factors, such as age, diet, use of other drugs, comorbidities, genetic polymorphisms, and vitamin K intake [3].

Compliance with OAC treatment is defined as the patient's state of agreement through the recommendations given by the clinician regarding this treatment, respecting the hours, dosage, frequency, and duration of prescription drugs [4].

There are countless factors that lead to patients not complying with this treatment such as numerous trips to the hospital, as well as the waiting time for consultation, their pathology, drug interactions, and personal beliefs. Thus, therapeutic doses are sometimes altered or interrupted by the patient [4].

The specific objective of this research topic was to describe and verify whether there is a relationship between patient compliance with OAC and patient gender and age. The gender and age group with the greatest adherence to OAC therapy was verified.

2. Materials and Methods

In this study, a descriptive–correlational, cross-sectional methodology was followed. A convenience sample was created with 111 participants. The data were collected from a questionnaire (validated through a pretest) completed by users of a hospital in Greater

Lisbon. In this study, a 90% confidence interval, an error of 10%, and a significance level of 0.1 were used. The responses were collected from users who attended a hypocoagulation consultation between 20 January 2020 and 20 February 2020.

In order to measure the adherence/compliance, an indirect method was used on the basis of responses to seven questions that investigated different situations potentially leading to nonadherence to therapy (failure to take OAC, failure to take OAC at the correct time, interruption of OAC due to improving symptoms, interruption of OAC due to worsening symptoms, compensation for missed OAC the previous day, interruption of therapy due to a lack of medication, and interruption of therapy according to the patient's initiative).

Patients provided their consent using a specific form, and the study was approved by the ethics committee of the hospital in question.

3. Results and Discussion

Of the 111 participants, 62.14% were female and 37.84% were male, with an age range of 19 to 87 years old. Great compliance was found with OAC therapy (98.20%), whereby only two male cases did not comply with correct therapy. It has been reported that the age group with the highest compliance was 71–80 years.

Regarding the specific questions in the questionnaire related to treatment adherence/compliance, the most answered option was "never". Specifically, 59.5% of patients had never failed to take OAC, 88.3% had never missed the exact hour, 96.4% had never interrupted OAC due to improving symptoms, 92.8% had never interrupted OAC due to worsening symptoms, 93.7% had never overcompensated following a missed previous dosage, 92.8 had never interrupted OAC due to a lack of medication, and 92.8% had never interrupted OAC according to their own initiative.

We found a significant and positive correlation between the variables "gender" and "compliance with OAC therapy", with $p\ (0.068) < \alpha\ (0.1)$, whereas there was a significant negative correlation between the variables "age by class" and "adherence to OAC therapy", with $p\ (0.091) < \alpha\ (0.1)$.

Institutional Review Board Statement: Ethical review and approval were waived for this study, due to high interest of cientific committee that asked the authors to conduct this specific study.

References

1. Silva, M.; Sousa, E.; Marques, F. Estado da arte na terapêutica anticoagulante: Novas abordagens. *Acta Farm. Port* **2013**, *2*, 5–18.
2. Barreira, R.; Ribeiro, F.; Martins, M. Monitorização da terapêutica com anticoagulantes orais: Consulta de anticoagulação vs. médico assistente. *Acta Med. Port* **2004**, *17*, 416–417.
3. Guimarães, J.; Zago, A. Anticoagulação Ambulatorial. *Rev. HCPA* **2007**, *27*, 30–38.
4. Ávila, C.; Aliti, B.; Feijó, M. Adesão farmacológica ao anticoagulante oral e os fatores que influenciam na estabilidade do índice de normatização internacional. *Rev. Lat. Am. Enf.* **2011**, *19*, 18–25. [CrossRef]

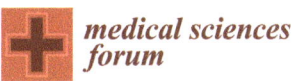

Proceeding Paper

S. aureus and MRSA Nasal Carriage in Dental Students: A Comprehensive Approach †

Patrícia Cavaco-Silva [1,*], Maria Mole [2], Beatriz Meliço [2] and Helena Barroso [1]

1. Centro de Investigação Interdisciplinar Egas Moniz (CiiEM), Instituto Universitário Egas Moniz, 2829-511 Almada, Portugal; mhbarroso@egasmoniz.edu.pt
2. Instituto Universitário Egas Moniz, 2829-511 Almada, Portugal; mariaanamole@gmail.com (M.M.); bia.melico.97@gmail.com (B.M.)
* Correspondence: montezpat@gmail.com
† Presented at the 5th International Congress of CiiEM—Reducing Inequalities in Health and Society, Online, 16–18 June 2021.

Abstract: *Staphylococcus aureus* and MRSA are important clinical pathogens representing a serious public health problem. This study aimed to determine the prevalence of *S. aureus* and methicillin-resistant *S. aureus* (MRSA) nasal carriage among dental students, identify the factors that influence this carriage, and characterize MRSA. A prevalence of *S. aureus* and MRSA carriage of 25.2% and 0.86% was estimated, respectively, and *SCCmec* Type VI, was identified in all isolated MRSA. The low MRSA colonization rate can reflect good infection control practices followed by students.

Keywords: *S. aureus*; MRSA; nasal carriage; dental students

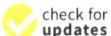

1. Introduction

Staphylococcus aureus is an important pathogen and carriage prevalence differs between populations. In dental practice, *S. aureus* transmission can occur between patients and dentists, and from contaminated surfaces and materials used during medical appointments. Therefore, monitorization of the presence of *S. aureus*, namely methicillin-resistant *S. aureus* (MRSA), in the dentistry teaching setting is important for the effective acquisition of infection and antibiotic resistance control practices [1].

2. Materials and Methods

A cross-sectional study was conducted in 2018 at a Dentistry University in the Lisbon Metropolitan Area, Portugal, to evaluate the prevalence of *S. aureus*/MRSA in dental students. Self-collected nasal swab specimens were obtained and bacterial isolates were identified using Mannitol Salt Agar, a MRSA chromogen agar and coagulase test. MRSA were confirmed with Mueller-Hinton agar/6 μg/mL oxacillin/4% NaCl and cefoxitin disk diffusion test. Epidemiological molecular characterization of MRSA was performed using a multiplex PCR assay for typing of Staphylococcal cassette chromosome *mec* (*SCCmec*), important for the identification and definition of MRSA clones [2]. Data were analyzed by using descriptive and inferential methodologies; a significance level of 5% was set in the latter case.

Ethics Committee Statement

The study was conducted according to the guidelines of the Declaration of Helsinki, and approved by the Ethics Committee of Egas Moniz (protocol code 668; date of approval: 28 November 2018).

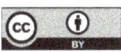

3. Results and Discussion

3.1. Prevalence of S. aureus and MRSA Nasal Carriage in Dental Students and Risk Factors

A sample of 464 students was obtained representing 55.4% of all dental students; 117 students were colonized with *S. aureus* and 4 had MRSA isolates, thus, a prevalence of *S. aureus* and MRSA carriage of 25.2% and 0.86% was estimated, respectively. A significative statistical relationship was found between curricular year and *S. aureus* carriage ($p = 0.05$), showing a higher colonization rate by 4th year students. A significative relation ($p = 0.024$) was also found between previous surgery and *S. aureus* colonization ($p = 0.008$). Additionally, male students were significantly more colonized than females ($p = 0.037$).

SCCmec Type VI was identified in all 7 MRSA isolates (four positive students) (Figure 1). *SCCmec* Type VI, characteristic of some MRSA clones normally associated with community infections, although less described in similar studies, matches the fact these students are starting their clinical practice [2].

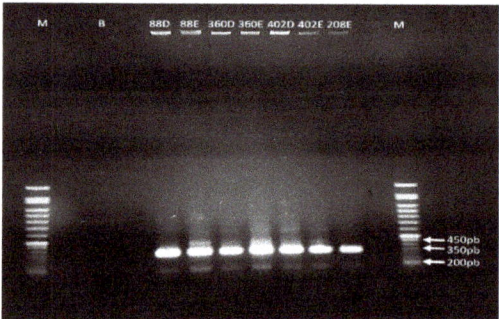

Figure 1. Agarose gel electrophoresis of products amplified by *SCCmec* multiplex PCR; 7 MRSA isolates from the 4 positive students (both left and right nasal cavities, except one student).

3.2. Molecular Characterization of MRSA Isolates

The estimated prevalence of *S. aureus* and MRSA is lower than found in other studies [1]. The higher *S. aureus* colonization rate by 4th grade students may be justified by their first contact with patients in the clinic. The higher *S. aureus* colonization rate in male students is also common [3]. The low colonization rate of MRSA (0.86%) can reflect good infection control practices followed by students. Additional studies would be interesting to characterize colonization patterns throughout Dentistry courses.

Informed Consent Statement: Informed consent was obtained from all subjects involved in the study.

Acknowledgments: The authors greatly thank the support of Egas Moniz teachers and students, without which this study would not have been possible.

Conflicts of Interest: The authors declare no conflict of interest.

References

1. Roberts, M.C.; Soge, O.O.; Horst, J.A.; Ly, K.A.; Milgrom, P. Methicillin-resistant Staphylococcus aureus from dental school clinic surfaces and students. *Am. J. Infect. Control* **2011**, *39*, 628–632. [CrossRef] [PubMed]
2. Lee, A.S.; de Lencastre, H.; Garau, J.; Kluytmans, J.; Malhotra-Kumar, S.; Peschel, A.; Harbarth, S. Methicillin-resistant *Sthaphylococcus aureus*. *Nat. Rev. Dis. Primers* **2018**, *4*, 18033. [CrossRef] [PubMed]
3. Olsen, K.; Sangvik, M.; Simonsen, G.S.; Sollid, J.U.E.; Sundsfjord, A.; Thune, I.; Furberg, A.S. Prevalence and population structure of *Staphylococcus aureus* nasal carriage in healthcare workers in a general population. The Tromsø Staph and Skin Study. *Epidemiol. Infect.* **2013**, *141*, 143–152. [CrossRef] [PubMed]

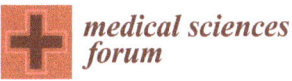

Proceedings

External Approach to Bilaterally Septated Maxillary Sinuses: A Case Report [†]

Pedro Gameiro *, Bernardo Saldanha, Francisco Santos, Jéssica Silva, João Norte, João Reis, Pedro Sottomayor, Rodolfo Vaz and Pedro Rodrigues

Egas Moniz's Dental Clinic Implantology Consultation, 2829-511 Caparica, Portugal; bernardopereira7@hotmail.com (B.S.); franciscosantos.em@gmail.com (F.S.); jessicasmsilva.md@gmail.com (J.S.); joaonorte7@gmail.com (J.N.); joao96reis@gmail.com (J.R.); pedro.rs.sottomayor@gmail.com (P.S.); rodolfovaz94@gmail.com (R.V.); pmsilvarodrigues@gmail.com (P.R.)
* Correspondence: pedrogilgameiro@gmail.com; Tel.: +351-91-446-8603
[†] Presented at the 5th International Congress of CiiEM—Reducing Inequalities in Health and Society, Online, 16–18 June 2021.

Abstract: The careful planning of a sinus lift procedure is the key to avoiding surgical complications. In this clinical case, a female patient, 59 years old and totally edentulous in the maxilla, was referred to Egas Moniz's Dental Clinic Implantology consultation with indication for bilateral external sinus lift of the maxillary sinuses prior to implant placement. Both orthopantomography and cone-beam computed tomography were used to show the anatomy of the maxillary sinuses, which presented multiple sinus septa. A multiple anterolateral window approach was applied in order to avoid perforation of the Schneiderian membrane while accessing it.

Keywords: sinus septa; maxillary sinus; Schneiderian membrane; external elevation of the maxillary sinus; oral surgery

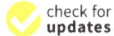

Citation: Gameiro, P.; Saldanha, B.; Santos, F.; Silva, J.; Norte, J.; Reis, J.; Sottomayor, P.; Vaz, R.; Rodrigues, P. External Approach to Bilaterally Septated Maxillary Sinuses: A Case Report. *Med. Sci. Forum* **2021**, *5*, 35. https://doi.org/10.3390/msf2021005035

Published: 22 July 2021

Publisher's Note: MDPI stays neutral with regard to jurisdictional claims in published maps and institutional affiliations.

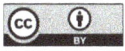

Copyright: © 2021 by the authors. Licensee MDPI, Basel, Switzerland. This article is an open access article distributed under the terms and conditions of the Creative Commons Attribution (CC BY) license (https://creativecommons.org/licenses/by/4.0/).

1. Introduction

An external maxillary sinus lift is a delicate surgical procedure that is performed when there is not enough bone available to allow implant placement in the posterior maxilla due to bone resorption of the alveolar process and pneumatization of the maxillary sinuses [1]. In order not to perforate the Schneiderian membrane, it is necessary to have full knowledge of the individual's maxillary sinus anatomy [2]. The literature shows the relationship between the presence of sinus septa and perforation of the Schneiderian membrane during surgery for external elevation of the maxillary sinus [2]. The location of the access varies according to the morphology and anatomical location of the septa [2].

2. Materials and Methods

A female patient, 59 years old and totally edentulous in the maxilla, was referred for consultation at the Egas Moniz's Dental Clinic Implantology with indication for bilateral external elevation of the maxillary sinuses. Orthopantomography and a CBCT (cone-beam computed tomography) scan revealed the presence of bilateral sinus septa in the anterolateral wall, resulting in its compartmentalization. Multiple accesses were performed for each sinus according to the anatomical position of each septum.

3. Results and Discussion

The same surgical approach was applied in both right and left maxillary sinuses. A full-thickness mucoperiosteal flap was executed at first, followed by an osteotomy using a round handpiece burr to gain sinus membrane access, creating two windows. Both access windows were elevated and the Schneiderian membrane was then detached. Both spaces were filled with xenograft Bio-Oss® and then covered with a Bio-Guide® collagen membrane. Orthopantomography and CBCT were performed after this procedure to check its final outcome. Multiple accesses allowed elevation of the maxillary sinus membranes with less risk of perforation (Figure 1).

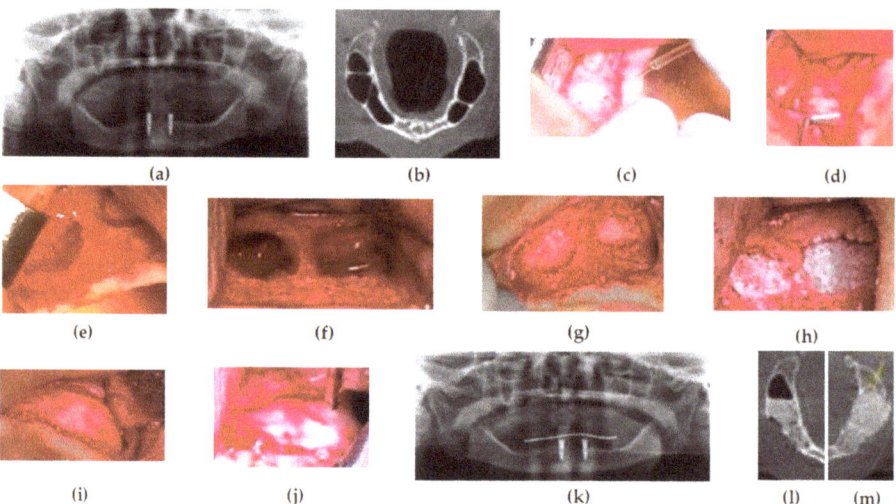

Figure 1. Surgical procedure: (**a**) initial orthopantomography; (**b**) initial CBCT scan; (**c**) osteotomy with round handpiece burr; (**d**) elevation of maxillary sinus access windows; (**e**) detached Schneiderian membrane on the right side; (**f**) detached Schneiderian membrane on the left side; (**g**) xenograft filling maxillary sinus access on the right side; (**h**) xenograft filling maxillary sinus access on the left side; (**i**) collagen membrane covering the graft on the right side; (**j**) collagen membrane covering the graft on the left side; (**k**) final orthopantomography; (**l**) final right-side CBCT scan; (**m**) final left-side CBCT scan.

In conclusion, septa should not be considered a contraindication to sinus lift surgery. Presurgical planning is crucial to reducing the risk of perforation of the Schneiderian membrane and enabling greater predictability of treatment success, thus reducing patient morbidity.

Institutional Review Board Statement: Not applicable.

Informed Consent Statement: Informed consent was obtained from all subjects involved in the study.

Conflicts of Interest: The authors declare no conflict of interest.

References

1. Tassos Irinakis, T.I.; Valentin Dabuleanu, V.D.; Salwa Aldahlawi, S.A. Complications during Maxillary Sinus Augmentation Associated with Interfering Septa: A New Classification of Septa. *Open Dent. J.* **2017**, *11*, 140–150. [CrossRef] [PubMed]
2. Magdalena Malec, M.M.; Tomasz Smektała, T.S.; Grzegorz Trybek, G.T.; Katarzyna Sporniak-Tutak, K.S. Maxillary sinus septa: Prevalence, morphology, diagnostics and implantological implications. Systematic review. *Folia Morphol.* **2014**, *73*, 259–266. [CrossRef]

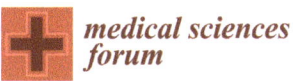

Proceeding Paper

Autologous Graft in the Anterior Maxilla—A Case Report †

Rodolfo Vaz *, Pedro Gameiro, Pedro Sottomayor, Bernardo Saldanha and Pedro Rodrigues

Implantology Consultation, Egas Moniz Dental Clinic, 2829-511 Almada, Portugal; pedrogilgameiro@gmail.com (P.G.); pedro.rs.sottomayor@gmail.com (P.S.); bernardopereira7@hotmail.com (B.S.); pmsilvarodrigues@gmail.com (P.R.)
* Correspondence: rodolfovaz94@gmail.com; Tel.: +351-914-084-902
† Presented at the 5th International Congress of CiiEM—Reducing Inequalities in Health and Society, Online, 16–18 June 2021.

Abstract: A 44-year-old male patient was referred to the Egas Moniz Dental Clinic, with a previous history of failed bone regeneration, resulting in a reduced buccal-palatal bone thickness and aesthetic compromise of the gingival margin of the anterior maxilla. Since the use of autologous bone is considered the "gold-standard" in guided bone regeneration, the treatment plan consisted of an autologous mental graft into the maxilla, with a simultaneous guided bone regeneration with a xenograft and absorbable membrane. This allowed a predictable volumetric bone regeneration with low patient morbidity and posterior fixed rehabilitation.

Keywords: autologous bone; bone graft; guided bone regeneration; implantology

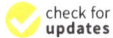

Citation: Vaz, R.; Gameiro, P.; Sottomayor, P.; Saldanha, B.; Rodrigues, P. Autologous Graft in the Anterior Maxilla—A Case Report. *Med. Sci. Forum* 2021, 5, 36. https://doi.org/10.3390/msf2021005036

Academic Editors: Helena Barroso and Cidália Castro

Published: 22 July 2021

Publisher's Note: MDPI stays neutral with regard to jurisdictional claims in published maps and institutional affiliations.

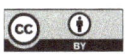

Copyright: © 2021 by the authors. Licensee MDPI, Basel, Switzerland. This article is an open access article distributed under the terms and conditions of the Creative Commons Attribution (CC BY) license (https://creativecommons.org/licenses/by/4.0/).

1. Introduction

Tooth extraction often leads to alveolar defects, which may present a difficult challenge to overcome, before the placement of implants, especially in the aesthetic zone. Depending on the size and location of the defect, different grafting materials can be used. Some materials, such as xenografts and allografts, and alloplastic materials of natural or synthetic origin, provide a scaffold, for new bone to grow. However, autogenous or autologous bone possesses osteoinductive, osteogenic, and osteoconductive properties, with a higher capacity of regeneration, when compared to other materials [1,2].

Various donor sites are available for autologous bone extraction. Regarding intraoral sites, the mandibular symphysis and the external oblique ridge of the mandible are the preferable donor sites, regarding both the quality and quantity of bone. Despite some potential complications described in the literature, as sensory alterations of the skin and mucosa, collection of bone from the symphysis provides thick and large grafts, suitable for vertical and horizontal augmentation [3,4].

Autologous bone is still considered the "gold standard" for bone augmentation, more importantly in cases of large and/or severe bone defects [2].

2. Materials and Methods

A 44-year-old male patient, without pathological and medicative references, and a regular smoker (about 10 cigarettes per day), was referred to the Egas Moniz Dental Clinic. Upon inspection, the patient presented a bone defect in the anterior maxilla on tooth #22, caused by a previous tooth extraction, and subsequent failed bone regeneration, which resulted in a reduced buccal-palatal bone thickness and aesthetic compromise of the gingival margin. Upon evaluation of the orthopantomography and CBCT scan, the treatment plan, which consisted of an autologous mental graft into the maxilla in conjunction with guided bone regeneration with a xenograft and absorbable membrane, was proposed to the patient and accepted.

3. Results and Discussion

After initial documentation, the first part of the surgery involved the exposure of the defect with a full thickness mucoperiosteal flap and measurement, facilitating the harvesting of bone.

Using the same method, the donor site was exposed, and an osteotomy was performed on the left mental region, to remove the bone block. Afterward, hemostasis was achieved, and the donor site was regenerated with collagen membrane and xenograft and sutured (Figure 1).

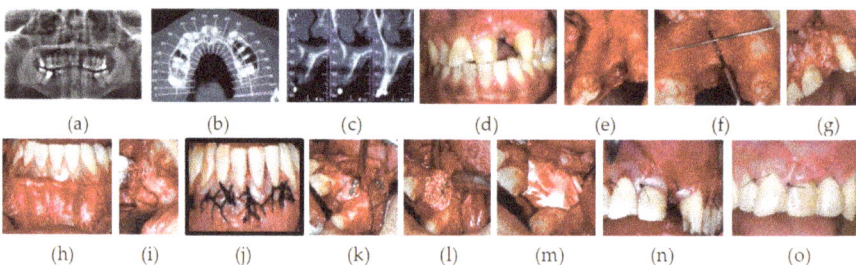

Figure 1. Surgical stages: (**a**) Orthopantomography; (**b**) CBCT scan (axial plane); (**c**) CBCT scan (sagittal plane); (**d**) initial photograph; (**e**) exposure of the defect; (**f**) measurements; (**g**) cortical perforations; (**h**) exposure of the donor site; (**i**) osteotomy; (**j**) suture of the donor site; (**k**) fixation of the bone block; (**l**) xenograft application; (**m**) collagen membrane placement; (**n**) suture of the recipient site; (**o**) provisional crown (1-week post-op).

Lastly, the bone block was held in place in the recipient site with fixation screws. A xenograft material (NanoBone®) was used to fill the rest of the defect, and an absorbable collagen membrane (Evolution OsteoBiol®) was applied, covering the bone grafting materials. The recipient site was then sutured. A provisional crown was lastly adhered to the adjacent teeth.

Due to the multi-dimensional defect present, the use of an autologous bone block was crucial, both to stabilize the grafting materials, as well as to ensure the maximum regenerative ability both vertically and in buccal-palatal thickness, thus confirming, that the use of autologous bone in large bone defects remains one of the best options for bone augmentation procedures.

Institutional Review Board Statement: Not applicable.

Informed Consent Statement: Informed consent was obtained from all subjects involved in the study.

Conflicts of Interest: The authors declare no conflict of interest.

References

1. Danesh-Sani, S.; Engebretson, S.; Janal, M. Histomorphometric results of different grafting materials and effect of healing time on bone maturation after sinus floor augmentation: A systematic review and meta-analysis. *J. Periodont Res.* **2016**, *52*, 301–312. [CrossRef] [PubMed]
2. Khoury, F.; Hanser, T. Mandibular Bone Block Harvesting from the Retromolar Region: A 10-Year Prospective Clinical Study. *Int. J. Oral Maxillofac. Implants* **2015**, *30*, 688–697. [CrossRef] [PubMed]
3. Reininger, D.; Cobo-Vazquez, C.; Monteserin-Matesanz, M.; Lopez-Quiles, J. Complications in the use of the mandibular body, ramus and symphysis as donor sites in bone graft surgery. A systematic review. *Medicina Oral Patologia Oral y Cirugia Bucal.* **2016**, *21*, 241–249. [CrossRef] [PubMed]
4. Pourabbas, R.; Nezafati, S. Clinical results of localized alveolar ridge augmentation with bone grafts harvested from symphysis in comparison with ramus. *J. Dent. Res. Dent. Clin. Dent. Prospect.* **2007**, *1*, 7–12. [CrossRef]

Proceeding Paper

Temporomandibular Disorders and Bruxism Prevalence in a Portuguese Sample [†]

João Belo [1], André Almeida [2,3], Paula Moleirinho-Alves [3] and Catarina Godinho [4,*]

1. Aluno do 5° ano do MIMD, Instituto Universitário Egas Moniz, 2829-511 Almada, Portugal; joaopbelo12@gmail.com
2. Centro de Investigação Interdisciplinar Egas Moniz, Egas Moniz—Cooperativa de Ensino Superior CRL, 2829-511 Almada, Portugal; andremarizalmeida@gmail.com
3. Hospital Cuf Tejo, 1350-352 Lisbon, Portugal; paula.m.alves@cuf.pt
4. Grupo de Patologia Médica, Nutrição e Exercício Clínico (PaMNEC), Centro de Investigação Interdisciplinar Egas Moniz, 2829-511 Almada, Portugal
* Correspondence: cgodinho@egasmoniz.edu.pt
† Presented at the 5th International Congress of CiiEM—Reducing Inequalities in Health and Society, Online, 16–18 June 2021.

Abstract: Temporomandibular disorder (TMD) encompasses a set of disorders involving the masticatory muscles, the temporomandibular joint and associated structures. It is a complex biopsychosocial disorder with several triggering, predisposing and perpetuating factors. In the etiology of TMD, oral parafunctions, namely bruxism, play a relevant role. The study of bruxism is complicated by some taxonomic and diagnostic aspects that have prevented achieving an acceptable standardization of diagnosis. The aim of this study was to analyze the prevalence of temporomandibular disorders and bruxism in a Portuguese sample.

Keywords: temporomandibular disorders; bruxism; awake bruxism; sleep bruxism

1. Introduction

Temporomandibular disorder (TMD) encompasses a set of disorders involving the masticatory muscles, the temporomandibular joint (TMJ) and associated structures [1]. The prevalence of painful TMD is about 10% in adults. It is a complex biopsychosocial disorder with several triggering, predisposing and perpetuating factors (macro- or micro-traumas, genetic, epigenetic, environmental, psychological and behavioral). In TMD etiology, oral parafunctions, namely bruxism, play a relevant role [2]. The definition of bruxism has undergone a constant evolution, currently being described as a repetitive and involuntary activity of the masticatory muscles, which is characterized by clenching or grinding of the teeth and/or by bracing (fixing) or thrusting (boosting) of the mandible, with or without dental contact [2].

2. Materials and Methods

An online questionnaire was applied using social networks as well as email contacts provided by the researchers. The questionnaire was translated to Portuguese based on a previous study [2]. This questionnaire included questions related to the characterization of TMD and bruxism (awake and sleep), as well as relevant medical history. Data were analyzed by descriptive methodology.

3. Results and Discussion

We obtained 256 answers to the questionnaire, consisting of responses from 196 females (76.56%) and from participants aged 18–24 (20.70%), 25–34 (21.88%), 35–54 (43.75%), 55–74 (12.11%) and +75 (1.56%). In Table 1, we can see the results obtained.

Table 1. TMD and bruxism in a sample of a Portuguese population.

Question	Yes	No
Have you ever had pain in your jaw, temple, ear, or in front of your ear on either side?	110 (42.9%)	145 (56.6%)
In the last 30 days, have you had any headaches, which include the area of the fountains in your head?	127 (49.6%)	129 (50.3%)
In the last 30 days, have you had any joint sound (or sounds) when you moved or used your jaw?	98 (38.2%)	158 (61.7%)
During the waking period, do you realize that you grind your teeth?	40 (15.6%)	215 (83.9%)
During the waking period, do you realize that you squeeze your teeth?	142 (55.4%)	114 (44.5%)
During the waking period do you realize that you push/press the jaw?	93 (36.3%)	163 (63.6%)
Has anyone informed you, or realized, that you grind your teeth or press your jaw during sleep?	98 (38.2%)	158 (61.7%)
If you wake up during sleep, do you usually experience discomfort in the lateral muscles areas of the face and/or head (masticatory muscles)?	70 (27.3%)	186 (72.6%)
In the last six months, have you had orofacial pain?	76 (29.6%)	180 (70.3%)

The key point to discuss is that more than half of the respondents did not notice pain in the jaw, in the temple area, in the ear or in front of the ear on both sides; they also did not notice any joint sound when they moved or used the jaw. As for awake bruxism, more than half of the respondents do not push/press the jaw. On the other hand, regarding the perception of clenching their teeth during the day, the vast majority responded positively. As far as sleep bruxism is concerned, more than half of the respondents stated that they do not notice grinding, pressing their teeth or feeling any discomfort in the muscle areas of the face and/or head (masticatory muscles). Similarly, with a significant difference, the respondents reported that they had no feeling of any kind of orofacial pain in the last 6 months.

Thus, we can conclude that although the values appear to be low regarding the prevalence of temporomandibular dysfunctions and bruxism in the Portuguese population, we have higher numbers compared with those in published studies [3].

Conflicts of Interest: The authors declare no conflict of interest.

References

1. Leeuw, R.; Klasser, G.D. *Orofacial Pain: Guidelines for Assessment, Diagnosis and Management*; Quintessence Books: Berlin, Germany, 2013.
2. Verhoeff, M.C.; Lobbezoo, F.; Wetselaar, P.; Aarab, G.; Koutris, M. Parkinson's disease, temporomandibular disorders and bruxism: A pilot study. *J. Oral Rehabil.* **2018**, *45*, 854–863. [CrossRef] [PubMed]
3. Almeida, A.; Cebola, P.; Manso, C.; Félix, S.; Maurício, P.; González, J.R. Prevalence of dysfunctional tempormandibular pathology and added jaw pain in periodical occupational medicine consultation at a Private Portuguese Health Services. *Ann. Med.* **2020**, *51* (Suppl. S1), 121. [CrossRef]

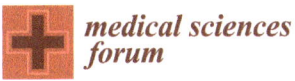

Proceeding Paper

Massive Testing Is Important to Control a SARS-CoV-2 Outbreak [†]

Daniela Guerreiro [1], Ana Luísa Costa [1], Teresa Nascimento [2,3], Ana Clara Ribeiro [2], Luís Proença [2], José João Mendes [2] and Helena Barroso [2,*]

[1] Instituto Universitário Egas Moniz (IUEM), 2829-511 Caparica, Portugal; daniela.guerreiro96@gmail.com (D.G.); analuisa.costa315@gmail.com (A.L.C.)
[2] Centro de Investigação Interdisciplinar Egas Moniz (CiiEM), Instituto Universitário Egas Moniz (IUEM), 2829-511 Caparica, Portugal; tnascimento@egasmoniz.edu.pt (T.N.); acribeiro@egasmoniz.edu.pt (A.C.R.); lproenca@egasmoniz.edu.pt (L.P.); jmendes@egasmoniz.edu.pt (J.J.M.)
[3] Unidade de Microbiologia Médica, Global Health and Tropical Medicine (GHTM), Instituto de Higiene e Medicina Tropical/Universidade Nova de Lisboa, 1349-008 Lisbon, Portugal
* Correspondence: mhbarroso@egasmoniz.edu.pt; Tel.: +351-21-294-6725
[†] Presented at the 5th International Congress of CiiEM—Reducing Inequalities in Health and Society, Online, 16–18 June 2021.

Abstract: At the end of September 2020, an outbreak of SARS-CoV-2 occurred at a university student's residence. A rapid response, with massive testing, using both RT-PCR and antigen rapid testing, helped to control the spread of the virus, showing the importance of tracking the infection. Testing for antibodies one month after the outbreak showed that the permanence of students with no infection in the same building was not a preponderant factor to develop an immune response.

Keywords: SARS-CoV-2; COVID-19; infection; immunological response

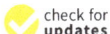

1. Introduction

On March 2020, the World Health Organization (WHO) communicated that due to its severity and alarming levels of spread, COVID-19 would be characterized as a pandemic [1]. With an increasing number of deaths, several countries have adopted the approach to massively screen the general population combined with contact tracing in an attempt to control the COVID-19 spread [2]. RT-PCR is the current standard for the diagnosis of acute COVID-19 for oral, nasal, or nasopharyngeal samples. However, rapid testing is emerging as the demand to screen large amounts of people in the shortest amount of time possible increases. Serology tests do not directly diagnose the presence of the virus, but the immune system molecules produced by the body as a response to the virus, such as IgM and IgG. These tests could play a major role in the fight against the current pandemic by accurately classifying the individuals who developed an immune response to SARS-CoV-2 [2]. Instituto Universitário Egas Moniz (IUEM) has on its grounds a university students' residence that accommodates young people from various nationalities, where epidemiological surveillance is constant. This work describes how a SAR-CoV-2 outbreak in the residence was controlled and characterizes the antibody response in students who remained confined.

2. Materials and Methods

Antigen rapid test devices (Panbio™ COVID-19), using nasopharyngeal swabs, were used to achieve massive testing of students and staff. During the outbreak, RT-PCR assays (GeneFinder Covid-19 Plus RealAmp Kit) were used to test students who contacted COVID-19 positive cases. Antibody rapid test device kits (Panbio™ IgG/IgM), using fingerstick blood, were used to assess the presence of SARS-CoV-2 antibodies in the residence's population. Informed consent of the participants was obtained.

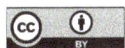

3. Results and Discussion

In September 2020, all students staying at the residence (165) and employees (22) (cleaning and security staff) were tested with an Ag rapid test device. No SARS-CoV-2 infection was detected. Two weeks after, it was known that one external student who attend a party was infected with SARS-CoV-2. Following this information all students at the residence that attended the party were tested for the presence of SARS-CoV-2 by RT-PCR assay. Four students were detected as positive for the virus. Then, all the remaining residents and staff were tested with an Ag rapid test device. Another three students were detected as positive. No member of staff tested positive. Five days after, two students who tested negative presented some symptoms related to COVID-19. They were retested and were positive. All positive students (9) were allocated to bedrooms situated in a specific area of the residence apart from the rest. All the others stayed in quarantine. During the next 14 days, students who stayed at the residence were not allowed to leave. At the end of the quarantine, all students, except two (the ones that became positive later), tested negative for SARS-CoV-2.

One month later, all students present at the residence and staff (142) were tested for antibodies using a rapid test device. IgG was detected in one member of the staff and in 20 students, 7 of which were students that tested positive during the outbreak and two students who had tested positive back in June and July 2020. Of note, in one student that had been positive in June, IgG was not detected. From the 132 students and staff with no previous known infection (with two or more negative tests), 48 stayed at the residence during quarantine and 84 were at their homes, with IgG-positive rates of 8.3% and 9.4% for both groups, respectively.

The two previously detected cases (June and July) indicated that antibodies can remain active for approximately 5 months, as others have already stated [3], although further studies are needed. Taking this into account, the 12 people that presented IgG and never tested positive could have possibly been infected, albeit asymptomatic, between July and October (not having tested positive in September) and were able to develop immunological responses.

This was a unique situation of an outbreak that arose in a university residence, a contained environment, where it was possible to observe, report, monitor, and verify the evolution of SARS-CoV-2 infection, evidencing that massive and timely testing is important to contain an outbreak. For people who never tested positive and developed an antibody response, no association was found between the place where the quarantine was fulfilled and being IgG detectable, showing that students' cohabitation in the same building was not a preponderant factor for developing an immunological response.

Institutional Review Board Statement: Ethical review and approval were waived for this study, due to the fact that this study was based on laboratory routine results of Covid detection and performed according the demand of national authorities of health in a pandemic context.

Informed Consent Statement: Informed consent was obtained from all subjects involved in the study.

Acknowledgments: Authors thank funding by CiiEM, Egas Moniz, Cooperativa de Ensino Superior, CRL.

Conflicts of Interest: The authors declare no conflict of interest.

References

1. General's Opening Remarks at the Media Briefing on COVID-19. 11 March 2020. Available online: https://www.who.int/director-general/speeches/detail/who-director-general-s-opening-remarks-at-the-media-briefing-on-covid-19---11-march-2020 (accessed on 22 March 2020).
2. Suhandynata, R.T.; Hoffman, M.A.; Kelner, M.J.; McLawhon, R.W.; Reed, S.L.; Fitzgerald, R.L. Longitudinal Monitoring of SARS-CoV-2 IgM and IgG Seropositivity to Detect COVID-19. *J. Appl. Lab. Med.* **2020**, *5*, 908–920. [CrossRef]
3. Wheatley, A.K.; Juno, J.A.; Wang, J.J.; Selva, K.J.; Reynaldi, A.; Tan, H.X.; Lee, W.S.; Wragg, K.M.; Kelly, H.G.; Esterbauer, R.; et al. Evolution of immune responses to SARS-CoV-2 in mild-moderate COVID-19. *Nat. Commun.* **2021**, *12*, 1162. [CrossRef] [PubMed]

Proceeding Paper

Detection of the SARS-CoV-2 UK Variant in Portugal [†]

Susana Bandarra [1,*], Lurdes Monteiro [1] and Laura Brum [2]

1. Molecular Pathology Laboratory, SYNLAB Lisboa, Av. Columbano Bordalo Pinheiro, 75 A, 1070-061 Lisbon, Portugal; lurdes.monteiro@synlab.pt
2. Clinical Laboratories SYNLAB Portugal, Av. Columbano Bordalo Pinheiro, 75 A, 1070-061 Lisbon, Portugal; laura.brum@synlab.pt
* Correspondence: susana.bandarra@synlab.pt
† Presented at the 5th International Congress of CiiEM—Reducing Inequalities in Health and Society, Online, 16–18 June 2021.

Abstract: At the end of 2020, a new highly transmissible variant of SARS-CoV-2 was discovered in the United Kingdom (UK). This work aims to identify potential cases of the UK variant in Portugal using routine diagnostic samples. A total of 26 out of 43 positive samples that were identified by RT-PCR as suspects were confirmed through sequencing to be the SARS-CoV-2 UK variant. The first case of the UK variant identified by us was in samples collected on 21 December 2020 at Lisbon airport in travelers from Manchester and London.

Keywords: SARS-CoV-2; COVID-19; Genomic epidemiology; UK variant; Spike mutation

1. Introduction

The SARS-CoV-2 strain lineage B.1.1.7, also known as the UK variant (or 501Y.V1), was identified as highly contagious in the UK. This variant, with the potential ability to evade host immunity [1,2], creates new challenges in the control of the pandemic, making the detection and tracking of this variant and others alike crucial to the long-term containment of SARS-CoV-2, mostly in the context of mass-vaccination. The early identification of B.1.1.7 in patients may help reducing further spread of this variant.

B.1.1.7 has a specific mutation in the Spike(S)-gene, which results in a deletion of two amino acids at sites 69 (histidine) and 70 (valine) (69–70 del) [3]. The multi-target design of some diagnostic tests that includes an S-gene target may function as a preliminary screening for the presence of mutations in S-gene, being a first clue of the B.1.1.7 lineage. Nevertheless, a confirmation is required by genome sequencing to achieve accurate results.

The sequencing of all SARS-CoV-2-positive cases is an expensive and time-consuming technique that requires samples with a high concentration of viral RNA and a high degree of purity to get satisfactory results. Public and private laboratories can play an important role in the early identification of B.1.1.7 or others by making an initial screening of the positive samples based in a simple RT-PCR diagnostic test and signaling the suspects for immediate confirmation. In this work, all the samples that had shown an absence of the S-gene in TaqPath COVID-19 diagnostic tests were considered as potentially being the UK variant.

2. Materials and Methods

Samples were obtained from routine diagnostics at SYNLAB Lisbon Laboratory. RNA was extracted from nasopharyngeal swabs and SARs-CoV-2 RNA detection was carried out through a multiplex real-time RT-PCR. Between December 21 (2020) and January 10 (2021), all positive samples, collected on the arrival area at International Lisbon Airport, were tested with a triple target assay, including S-gene target (Applied Biosystems TaqPath COVID-19 CE-IVD RT-PCR Kit), according to the manufacturer's instructions. In cases where S-gene was not detected but ORF1ab and N genes were amplified, RNA samples were sequenced and analyzed by the National Institute of Health (INSA) Doctor Ricardo Jorge, Portugal. The UK variant was also analyzed in the community using the same approach in random samples collected between 6 to 9 of January. Some of them were also sequenced.

This study was performed in accordance with the General-Directorate of Health (DGS) guidelines. Informed consent was obtained from all patients and all samples are obtained under the service-providing activity of the SYNLAB Health laboratory in the diagnostic area, and thus, the ethical procedures inherent in obtaining them are fully respected.

3. Results and Discussion

A screening of a total of 76 cases of SARS-CoV-2-positive travelers is summarized in Table 1.

Table 1. Identification of SARS-CoV-2 UK variant in travelers that arrived at Lisbon airport.

Positive Cases	S gene Dropout	Identified as S: N501Y.V1 UK
76	43 (56.6%)	26 (60.5%) [1]

[1] 17 cases not identified as 501Y.V1 without any NGS result associated.

Most of the analyzed samples were from British travelers. In total, 60.5% of the SARS-CoV-2-positive cases with S-gene dropout were confirmed by sequencing as being the UK variant (lineage B.1.1.7). It should be noted that of the 43 S-gene dropout samples, 17 could not be sequenced because of the RNA quality needed for sequencing. Curiously, one of the confirmed UK variant samples was identified in a traveler who departed from Chisinau, Moldova International Airport.

Two weeks after the first cases were identified, when applying the same methodology to random cases detected as positive in the community samples, we found that 11 of the 13 SARS-CoV-2 infection cases that showed S-gene dropout after being sequenced proved to be the UK variant. These samples were collected in Lisbon, Setubal, and Algarve. This suggests that the UK variant had a fast spread within the community. At this time, the lab screened around 558 samples for S-gene detection per day and it was observed that from 148 ± 33 positive cases, $16 \pm 3\%$ did not amplify the S-gene.

Given the high number of positive samples that need to be screened through genome sequencing to identify the UK variant, this work demonstrates the importance of using RT-PCR diagnostic tests in diagnostic laboratories as a preliminary screening tool for early signaling of potential UK variant cases before genome sequencing. This work also demonstrates the important role of private diagnostic laboratories in complementing the Public Institutions regarding the identification of highly spreading variants.

Institutional Review Board Statement: Ethical review and approval were waived for this study, due to the fact that this study was based on laboratory routine results of Covid detection and performed according the demand of national authorities of health in a pandemic context.

Informed Consent Statement: Informed consent was obtained from all subjects involved in the study.

Acknowledgments: We thank the Molecular Pathology Laboratory Lisbon team for the diagnosis work.

Conflicts of Interest: The authors declare no conflict of interest.

References

1. Davies, N.G.; Abbott, S.; Barnard, R.C.; Jarvis, C.I.; Kucharski, A.J.; Munday, J.D.; Pearson, C.A.; Russell, T.W.; Tully, D.C.; Washburne, A.D.; et al. Estimated transmissibility and impact of SARS-CoV-2 lineage B.1.1.7 in England. *Science* **2021**, *372*, abg3055. [CrossRef] [PubMed]
2. Cele, S.; Gazy, I.; Jackson, L.; Hwa, S.-H.; Tegally, H.; Lustig, G. Escape of SARS-CoV-2 501Y.V2 from neutralization by convalescent plasma. *Nature* **2021**, *593*, 142–146. [CrossRef] [PubMed]
3. Leung, K.; Shum, M.H.; Leung, G.M.; Lam, T.T.; Wu, J.T. Early transmissibility assessment of the N501Y mutant strains of SARS-CoV-2 in the United Kingdom. *Euro Surveill.* **2021**, *26*, 2002106. [CrossRef] [PubMed]

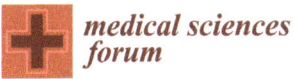

Proceeding Paper

Oral Health among Athletes at the Egas Moniz Sports Dentistry Practice †

Carolina Fernandes [1], Inês Allen [1], Leonor Sá Pinto [1], André Júdice [1,2], Filipa Vicente [1,3], Carlos Família [3,4], José João Mendes [1,2,3] and Catarina Godinho [1,3,*]

1. Sport Dentistry Consultation at Egas Moniz Dental Clinic, Instituto Universitário Egas Moniz, 2829-511 Almada, Portugal; carolinaf2801@gmail.com (C.F.); inesallen06@gmail.com (I.A.); nonosapinto@gmail.com (L.S.P.); judice87@gmail.com (A.J.); fvicente@egasmoniz.edu.pt (F.V.); jmendes@egasmoniz.edu.pt (J.J.M.)
2. Clinical Research Unit (CRU), Centro de Investigação Interdisciplinar Egas Moniz, 2829-511 Almada, Portugal
3. Medical Pathophysiology, Nutrition and Clinical Exercise Group (PaMNEC), Instituto Universitário Egas Moniz, 2829-511 Almada, Portugal; carlosfamilia@egasmoniz.edu.pt
4. Molecular Pathology Laboratory, Instituto Universitário Egas Moniz, 2829-511 Almada, Portugal
* Correspondence: cgodinho@egasmoniz.edu.pt
† Presented at the 5th International Congress of CiiEM—Reducing Inequalities in Health and Society, Online, 16–18 June 2021.

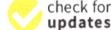

Abstract: The sports dentistry consultation at the Clínica Universitária Egas Moniz is guaranteed by a multidisciplinary team of health professionals that provide a customized service to high performance athletes. Over the last year, 99 athletes were evaluated in terms of their oral health through extraoral, intraoral and radiographic exams. In this population a high prevalence of dry mouth, erosive wear, gingivitis, periodontitis and DMF index was observed, which may have a profound and negative impact on sports performance. Of the athletes, 40.4% attended follow up consultations, where restoration and scaling were the majority of the clinical procedures performed. This data highlights the importance of a dedicated sports dentistry consultations.

Keywords: sport; athlete; athletic performance; sports dentistry; oral health; dental caries; dental erosion; periodontal disease; temporomandibular disorders

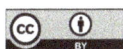

1. Introduction

Sports dentistry (SD) is an area whose main focus is the promotion of oral health and the prevention of orofacial injuries that might disrupt the athletes' performance [1]. Over the last decade the European Association for Sports Dentistry (EA4SD) and the Academy for Sports Dentistry (ASD) have reinforced the need to create stronger links between dentistry and sports, in order to guarantee the best health care for athletes of all ages, levels and modalities [2]. The practice of sports, especially in high performance athletes, has been shown to be affected by the needs of each individual, by their oral and systemic health and by their physical and psychological state [3]. Research shows that athletes' oral health is usually poor and careless, causing oral lesions that can quickly manifest themselves at the joint, muscular or even systemic levels [3]. Therefore, the dentist should be able to adequately attend the physical and psychological consequences of an injury, and determine the best strategy for the prevention, diagnosis and treatment of oral diseases, depending on the sports' modality [2]. With the present work we describe the overall oral health status of high-performance athletes followed at the sports dentistry consultation over the last year and reiterate the importance of the existence of such a consultation.

2. Materials and Methods

In this longitudinal observational study were included athletes who followed the sports dentistry consultation during the year of 2020, after providing informed consent.

Evaluation of the athletes' oral health began with triage, where extraoral, intraoral and radiographic examinations were performed. Demographic data (age, sex), data related to sports (modality), eating habits (added sugars), and hygiene habits (number of daily teeth brushings) were recorded. The presence of dry mouth, tooth decay and erosion, periodontal disease, temporomandibular disorders and third molars were also recorded. The presence of caries was evaluated through the DMF index (decayed, missing and filled). The presence of dental erosion was evaluated by sextants. Periodontal disease was reflected by the manifestation of gingivitis or periodontitis. Occlusal problems were assessed according to the presence of changes in the temporomandibular joint (TMJ).

3. Results and Discussion

This study included 99 athletes, of which 89.9% were male. The age of these athletes ranged between 16 and 60 years, and the large majority were dedicated to football (62.6%), athletics (7.1%) or basketball (5.1%). A large number of these athletes reported good oral hygiene habits, brushing their teeth more than twice a day (89.9%). Furthermore, 19.2% of the athletes reported feeling a dry mouth. Subsequent evaluation of the DMF index, showed that on average these athletes had 3.12 ± 2.8 decayed teeth, 0.821 ± 1.76 missing teeth and 3.75 ± 3.80 filled teeth, with an overall index of 7.28 ± 4.87. As for dental erosion, 27.9% showed erosive wear in at least one quadrant. Though the DMF index is lower than that previously reported for soccer players, the DMF index was higher for our sample [4]. Regarding periodontal disease, 37.4% presented gingivitis and 10.1% periodontitis. As for TMJ problems, 20.2% showed to have some type of joint disorder. This data shows that in general, athletes have more filled than decayed or missing teeth, have a high prevalence of dental erosion, gingivitis, periodontitis and TMJ problems, problems that need to be rapidly addressed, before further deterioration. Of these athletes, 40.4% attended follow up consultations, subsequent to triage, to address these problems, where restoration and scaling composed the majority of the clinical procedures performed (43.0% and 28.1%, respectively). With this study we show the importance of the establishment of dedicated sports dentistry consultations, that promote prevention, and allow the identification and subsequent treatment of oral pathologies in athletes, as these may have a profound and negative impact on their sports performance.

Institutional Review Board Statement: The study was conducted according to the guidelines of the Declaration of Helsinki, and approved by the Institutional Review Board of Egas Moniz, Cooperativa de Ensino Superior. Ethical review and approval were waived for this study, due to all users of the Egas Moniz Dental Clinic signed a consent form (given the educational nature of this clinic) at the time of their first visit (triage). This document was approved by all the institutional bodies responsible for education and research in this institution.

Informed Consent Statement: Informed consent was obtained from all subjects involved in the study.

Data Availability Statement: All available data are accessible in the central computer database of the Egas Moniz Dental Clinic.

Conflicts of Interest: The authors declare no conflict of interest.

References

1. Sousa, M.; Mendes, J.J.; Godinho, C. Medicina Dentária Desportiva: Ideologia ou Necessidade? *Proelium* **2016**, *7*, 135–164.
2. Stamos, A.; Mills, S.; Malliaropoulos, N.; Cantamessa, S.; Dartevelle, J.L.; Gündüz, E.; Laubmeier, J.; Hoy, J.; Kakavas, G.; Le Garrec, S.; et al. The European Association for Sports Dentistry, Academy for Sports Dentistry, European College of Sports and Exercise Physicians consensus statement on sports dentistry integration in sports medicine. *Dent. Traumatol.* **2020**, *36*, 1–5. [CrossRef] [PubMed]
3. Gallagher, J.; Ashley, P.; Petrie, A.; Oral, N.I. A running battle with oral diseases—Are we in with a sporting Here has been. *Braz. Dent. J.* **2020**, *227*, 370.
4. Needleman, I.; Ashley, P.; Meehan, L.; Petrie, A.; Weiler, R.; McNally, S.; Ayer, C.; Hanna, R.; Hunt, I.; Kell, S.; et al. Poor oral health including active caries in 187 UK professional male football players: Clinical dental examination performed by dentists. *Br. J. Sports Med.* **2016**, *50*, 41–44. [CrossRef]

Proceeding Paper

Study of the Phenolic Content and the Antioxidant Capacity of *Rubus idaeus* L. Genotypes within the Development of a National Cultivar [†]

Rita Cornamusaz [1], Francisco Luz [2], Pedro Brás de Oliveira [2], Margarida Moncada [3] and Madalena Bettencourt da Câmara [3,*]

1. Instituto Universitário Egas Moniz, 2829-511 Almada, Portugal; ritac.16@gmail.com
2. Instituto Nacional de Investigação Agrária e Veterinária, I.P. (INIAV, I.P.), 2784-505 Oeiras, Portugal; franciscorluz@hotmail.com (F.L.); pedro.oliveira@iniav.pt (P.B.d.O.)
3. Centro de Investigação Interdisciplinar Egas Moniz, CiiEM, Instituto Universitário Egas Moniz, 2829-511 Almada, Portugal; margaridacm@egasmoniz.edu.pt
* Correspondence: mbettencourt@egasmoniz.edu.pt
† Presented at the 5th International Congress of CiiEM—Reducing Inequalities in Health and Society, Online, 16–18 June 2021.

Abstract: The production of raspberries in Portugal has increased considerably in the last two decades, assuming a great economic interest today. Here, we studied the phenolic content and the antioxidant capacity of selected genotypes within a breeding program. The results suggest that this program may be unintentionally selecting raspberry phenolics. If so, this would be of particular interest, since there is scientific evidence that raspberry phenolics or their metabolites may have beneficial health effects, namely antioxidant activity.

Keywords: red raspberry; genotypes; cultivar selection; total phenols; antioxidant capacity

1. Introduction

Raspberry production in Portugal is currently of great economic interest, offering sustenance for small and large farmers. In 2018, the Instituto Nacional de Investigação Agrária e Veterinária, in close partnership with Beira Baga, an enterprise that produces and commercializes small fruits, started a small breeding program in order to release raspberry cultivars for all growers. This is particularly important when all raspberry cultivars are only released for exclusive or club growers. This study aims to investigate if the *Rubus idaeus* L. genotypes selected within the program by their agronomic and commercial quality parameters are also more abundant in phenolic compounds and have a higher antioxidant capacity.

2. Materials and Methods

The plants were installed in May 2019 at the Fataca Innovation Pole in Odemira, Portugal (planted in 36-l Styrofoam containers at a density of 3 plants per linear meter over tunnels covered in polyethylene plastic) (Figure 1a). All genotypes were fruitful in the first year of release in the fall. Production was recorded, and an empirical and expeditious survey of some of the most relevant quality characteristics of the fruit fresh and after 7 days stored at 4 °C, such as size, color/brightness and texture (Figure 1b). After this period, the genotypes best positioned in the hierarchy were selected. The laboratory work was carried out on samples of 12 genotypes, 9 red and 3 yellow raspberries (RRG and YRG), and 4 cultivars (Cv) of *Rubus idaeus* L. All samples were analyzed for their brix degree (NP EN 12143) and humidity content (Organization for Cooperation and Development method) [1]. A raspberry extract rich in phenolic compounds (extract solution composition—methanol:water:formic acid, 79.9:20:0.1 %v/v) [1] was made for 6 selected genotypes, 5 red and 1 yellow raspberries (RRG and YRG), and 4 cultivars (Cv) of *Rubus idaeus* L. in triplicate. Then, the extract content of the total phenols (TP) was determined by Folin–Ciocalteau [1], and their in vitro antioxidant capacity was measured by the Ferric-Reducing Antioxidant Power (FRAP) method [2].

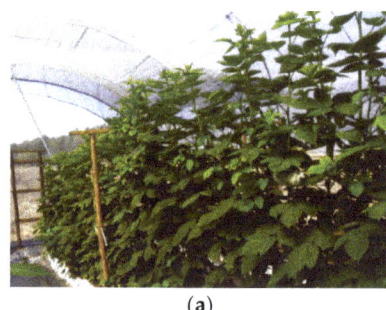 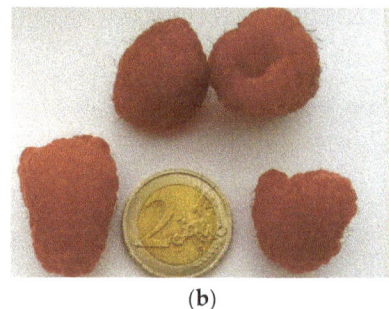

(a) (b)

Figure 1. Aspects of the plants' installation at Fataca Innovation Pole in Odemira, Portugal (**a**); quality evaluation aspects of fresh *Rubus idaeus* L. in the field for selection (**b**).

3. Results and Discussion

Generally, breeding programs aim to optimize plants and fruits for certain production systems, mainly based on parameters such as yield, capacity to resist pests and diseases, quality attributes such as the taste and texture of fruits or their ability to maintain their quality postharvest, among others. The phytochemical composition of raspberries is not currently a selection parameter. However, that composition depends on the genotype, among others factors.

This preliminary study evaluated aspects of the quality and composition and phytochemical activity of fruits of selected genotypes and cultivars, the latter for comparison purposes. The humidity and brix degrees obtained for all the samples varied, respectively, between 88.3% and 90.7% and 5.5° and 9.8°. The TP and FRAP contents (mg gallic acid eq. and Trolox eq. µmoles/100 g fresh fruit, respectively) of the selected samples were among 96.2–124.1 and 722.5–1011.1 (RRG), 104.7 and 899.3 (YRG) and 151.4–202.3 and 1113.6–1436.2 (Cv). The results of all the samples were within the values published for raspberries [1,3]. The findings obtained here seem to support the investigation question, as the four RRG selected in 2020 had higher TP contents than the rejected one. However, all Cv had higher TP and FRAP values. It is interesting to note that the selection made seemed to also take into consideration raspberry phenolics. These constituents are largely responsible for their antioxidant capacity and, according to scientific evidence, can also contribute to other beneficial health effects.

Institutional Review Board Statement: Not applicable.

Informed Consent Statement: Not applicable.

Data Availability Statement: Not applicable.

Conflicts of Interest: The authors declare no conflict of interest.

References

1. Correia, M. Caracterização Química e Avaliação da Atividade Biológica da Framboesa (*Rubus idaeus* L.): Contribuição para o Desenvolvimento de Uma Alegação de Saúde. Ph.D. Thesis, Universidade de Lisboa, Lisboa, Portugal, 2016.
2. Thaipong, K.; Boonprakoba, U.; Crosby, K.; Cisneros-Zevallosc, L.; Byrnec, D.H. Comparison of ABTS, DPPH, FRAP, and ORAC assays for estimating antioxidant activity from guava fruit extracts. *J. Food Compos. Anal.* **2006**, *19*, 669–675. [CrossRef]
3. García, A.V.; Pérez, S.E.M.; Butsko, M.; Moya, M.S.P.; Sanahuja, A.B. Authentication of "Adelita" Raspberry Cultivar Based on Physical Properties, Antioxidant Activity and Volatile Profile. *Antioxidants* **2020**, *9*, 593. [CrossRef] [PubMed]

Proceeding Paper

Effect of 6% Maltodextrin Intake on Capillary Lactate Concentration in Soccer Players [†]

Adinylson Fonseca [1], Maria Alexandra Bernardo [1,2], Maria Fernanda de Mesquita [1,2], José Brito [1,2] and Maria Leonor Silva [1,2,*]

1. Instituto Universitário Egas Moniz (IUEM), 2829-511 Almada, Portugal; adinylson@gmail.com (A.F.); abernardo@egasmoniz.edu.pt (M.A.B.); fmesquita@egasmoniz.edu.pt (M.F.d.M.); britojaa@hotmail.com (J.B.)
2. Centro de Investigação Interdisciplinar Egas Moniz (CiiEM), Instituto Universitário Egas Moniz, 2929-511 Almada, Portugal
* Correspondence: lsilva@egasmoniz.edu.pt
† Presented at the 5th International Congress of CiiEM—Reducing Inequalities in Health and Society, Online, 16–18 June 2021.

Abstract: Recent literature suggests that ergogenic substances may play a beneficial role in intermittent exercise. Maltodextrin supplementation has been investigated in soccer players, but few studies have been reported. The aim of this study was to evaluate the effect of 6% maltodextrin supplementation on capillary lactate in soccer players. The study was carried out during soccer training, which was characterised by intense activity (90 min). Participants (n = 24) were randomly allocated in control (water) and intervention (6% maltodextrin solution) groups. Capillary lactate levels were evaluated at pre-exercise (0 min—t0), exercise (45 min—t1), and post-exercise (90 min—t2) moments. At t1, the mean capillary lactate concentration value was significantly higher in players not supplemented with 6% maltodextrin (5.47 mmol/L) than in supplemented players (4.79 mmol/L).

Keywords: maltodextrin; carbohydrates; capillary lactate; soccer players

1. Introduction

Football is a sport with intermittent exercises of varying intensity. About 88% of the time of a football match involves aerobic activities, and 12% involves high-intensity anaerobic activities. Performance during intermittent sport is dependent upon the anaerobic and aerobic energy combination. High-intensity exercise implies a greater intramuscular accumulation of lactate, which may lead to extreme fatigue. The accumulation of lactate is one of the most important causes of skeletal muscle fatigue, i.e., a decline in muscle strength, which consequently leads to a decrease in exercise performance. Carbohydrates have been the most commonly used substrate as an ergogenic resource before sport, as it has been found that their intake in intermittent sport can have a positive impact on performance [1–3]. The aim of the present study was to evaluate the effect of 6% maltodextrin supplementation on capillary lactate concentration in soccer players.

2. Materials and Methods

Following Cooperativa Egas Moniz Ethical Committee approval, 24 male professional soccer players with ages between 18 and 35 years were recruited from three football clubs. After the collection of written informed consent, participants were randomly allocated in a control group (ingestion of 250 mL of water; n = 12) or an intervention group (ingestion of 250 mL of 6% maltodextrin solution; n = 12). The study was conducted during a regular soccer field practice (90 min). The intervention and control groups ingested, respectively, maltodextrin or water immediately before the soccer practice. Capillary lactate was evaluated in both groups at pre-exercise (t0), during exercise (45 min; t1), and post-exercise (90 min; t2) moments. At baseline, anthropometric and 24-h dietary recall data were taken for both groups. A mixed type, repeated measures ANOVA was used for statistical analysis at the 5% level of significance.

3. Results and Discussion

Results revealed that there was interaction between the independent and repeated measure factors ($F_{(1.31)}$ = 38.124; $p < 0.001$), which means that it was possible to infer differences in capillary lactate at different moments. At the t1 moment, the mean capillary lactate concentration value was significantly higher in players not supplemented with 6% maltodextrin (5.47 mmol/L) than in supplemented players (4.79 mmol/L). However, at the t2 moment, no significant differences were found between non-supplemented players (2.13 mmol/L) and maltodextrin-supplemented players (2.67 mmol/L) (Figure 1).

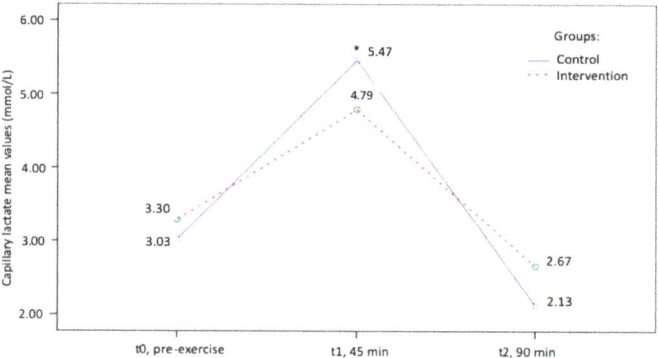

Figure 1. Mean soccer player capillary lactate values (mmol/L) in control (blue line) and intervention (red line) groups for the 3 studied moments: t_0, t_1 and t_2; (*)—the difference of mean capillary lactate concentration values between groups with statistical significance.

The two groups were considered homogeneous because there were no significant differences ($p < 0.05$) for the mean values of the anthropometric parameters of food intake (on the day before the intervention) and capillary lactate levels at t_0. Data of the present study showed that 6% maltodextrin supplementation decreased the mean capillary lactate values in a short time, which could mean an improvement of performance in the middle of a soccer game. These results were in agreement with those of previous studies in which maltodextrin did not reveal significant differences at a post-exercise moment, suggesting that maltodextrin did not increase glycogen content post-resistance exercise [4]. From this study, it can be concluded that the ingestion of 6% maltodextrin can play a beneficial role by decreasing the mean values of capillary lactate concentration in soccer players in the middle of a soccer game. These results may represent an important application in the performance of professional soccer players, since they are subject to intense training that is associated with fatigue. In this context, pre-exercise supplementation with maltodextrin may decrease lactate accumulation and consequently reduce fatigue.

Institutional Review Board Statement: The study was conducted according to the guidelines of the Declaration of Helsinki, and approved by the Ethical Committee of the Cooperativa de Ensino Egas Moniz (protocol code 619 and date of approval 30 May 2018).

Informed Consent Statement: Informed consent was obtained from all subjects involved in the study.

Data Availability Statement: Not applicable.

Acknowledgments: The authors thank the Biochemistry Laboratory of Cooperativa de Ensino Superior Egas Moniz and Master in Clinical Nutrition of Instituto Universitário Egas Moniz for support.

Conflicts of Interest: The authors declare no conflict of interest.

References

1. Fiorenza, M.; Hostrup, M.; Gunnarsson, T.; Shirai, Y.; Schena, F.; Iaia, F.; Bangsbo, J. Neuromuscular Fatigue and Metabolism during High-Intensity Intermittent Exercise. *Med. Sci. Sports Exerc.* **2019**, *51*, 1642–1652. [CrossRef] [PubMed]
2. Baker, L.; Rollo, I.; Stein, K.; Jeukendrup, A. Acute effects of carbohydrate supplementation on intermittent sports performance. *Nutrients* **2015**, *7*, 5733–5763. [CrossRef] [PubMed]
3. Stevenson, E.; Watson, A.; Theis, S.; Holz, A.; Harper, L.; Russell, M. A comparison of isomaltulose versus maltodextrin ingestion during soccer-specific exercise. *Eur. J. Appl. Physiol.* **2017**, *117*, 2321–2333. [CrossRef] [PubMed]
4. Wilburn, D.; Machek, S.; Cardaci, T.; Hwang, P.; Willoughby, D. Acute Maltodextrin Supplementation During Resistance Exercise. *J. Sports Sci. Med.* **2020**, *19*, 282–288. [PubMed]

Proceeding Paper

Influence of Maturation on Sports Injuries Profile in Portuguese Youth [†]

Lara Costa e Silva *[ ], Júlia Teles [ ] and Isabel Fragoso

CIPER, Faculty of Human Kinetics, University of Lisbon, 1495-751 Cruz Quebrada, Portugal; jteles@fmh.ulisboa.pt (J.T.); ifragoso@fmh.ulisboa.pt (I.F.)
* Correspondence: laras@uatlantica.pt
† Presented at the 5th International Congress of CiiEM—Reducing Inequalities in Health and Society, Online, 16–18 June 2021.

Abstract: Physical activity (PA) is beneficial, enhancing healthy development. However, it is estimated that one third of school-age children practicing sport regularly suffer from a serious injury. Maturation can make young athletes more vulnerable to sports injuries and increased knowledge about injury with specific PA exposure data is important to an overall risk management strategy. The aim of this study was to determine the influence of maturation on sports injury profiles in Portuguese youths. Distance to peak height velocity (PHV) was a significant predictor of injury patterns in children and adolescents of both sexes.

Keywords: injuries; children and adolescents; bone age; peak height velocity; physical activity level

1. Introduction

Musculoskeletal injuries are the most common injuries in youth sports. Growth spurts, maturity-associated variations, and a lack of complex motor skills needed for certain sports are among the risk factors that may play an important role in the growing athlete [1–3]. An epidemic of both acute and overuse injuries has been considered as children make the transition to adolescence. Enhanced environments for injury can occur and several authors have reported structural and tissue changes that may contribute to this situation [1–3]. As children and adolescents participate in sports in record numbers, targeting risk groups is important [3]. Therefore, our aim was to determine the influence of maturation on sports injury profiles of Portuguese youths.

2. Materials and Methods

The injury profiles and PA level information were obtained by LESADO and RAPIL II questionnaires. They were distributed to 651 participants aged between 10 and 18 years attending four schools. Maturity measures were evaluated through maturity offset (time before or after peak height velocity—PHV) and the Tanner-Whitehouse III method. Univariate analysis was used to identify the set of candidate predictors for the regression analysis that was used to determine significant predictors of injury occurrence, injury rate, injury type, and body area injury location. The Ethics Committee of the Faculty of Human Kinetics approved the research protocol. Before inclusion in the study all subjects' parents gave their written informed consent. STROBE guidelines were followed.

3. Results and Discussion

A total of 651 subjects participated in this study, aged between 10 and 18 years (Mean = 13.7 years; Standard Deviation = 1.8 years). A total of 247 subjects reported a sports injury during the previous six months (37.9%; 95% CI: 34.2–41.7%). Considering the analysis by sex, 42.1% of the boys and 33.9% of the girls reported an injury. The injury rate was 11.8 per 1000 h. Regarding predictors, the probability of injury increased approximately two times in girls who had already passed PHV ($p = 0.009$). Early mature girls ($p = 0.007$), with higher bone age ($p = 0.012$) and close to PHV ($p = 0.033$), showed a higher injury rate. Additionally, as maturity offset decreased, the chances of girls having a strain or a fracture increased 2 times ($\chi^2 (2) = 15.115$, $p = 0.001$). In boys, the probability of injury to the upper limbs was higher before PHV and in the lower limbs it was higher after PHV ($\chi^2 (2) = 6.014$, $p = 0.049$).

Some injury risk factors are unique to the growing athlete. Sports injury profiles in youths are significantly influenced by maturation [2]. Girls near PHV may be particularly vulnerable to sports injury risk due to the physiological processes of growth. An increase in traumatic injuries takes place mainly during the year of PHV, while the increase in overuse injuries persists in the year after PHV. Imbalance between strength and flexibility, joint stiffness, decreased bone density, and abnormal movement mechanics during the year of maximal growth contributes to an increase in traumatic injuries. Additionally if muscles, tendons, and apophyses adapt slowly, and activities are performed repetitively, those tissues are not immediately able to deal with the increased stress and overuse injuries may occur after PHV [4]. Body area injury location in boys is significantly different before and after PHV. Younger athletes are more likely to have bone fractures located in the upper limbs that are associated with traumatic injuries due to a transient decrease in coordination, balance, and complex motor skills [5]. On the other hand, increased stress occurs as the changes in the length, mass, and moment of inertia of the extremities take place with growth. These complex factors may be conducive to the development of overuse injuries, especially in lower limbs after PHV [6].

Due to the variation in timing of maturation, chronological age may not be an absolute indicator for injury risk and the assessment of maturation should be strongly encouraged.

Institutional Review Board Statement: The study was conducted according to the guidelines of the Declaration of Helsinki, and approved by the Ethics Committee of the Faculty of Human Kinetics, University of Lisbon (50/2015).

Informed Consent Statement: Informed consent was obtained from all subjects involved in the study.

Data Availability Statement: The data presented in this study are available on request from the corresponding author.

Acknowledgments: We would like to express our gratitude to Carlos Barrigas, Ana Silva, and João Albuquerque. Lara Costa e Silva, Ana Silva, and João Albuquerque were supported by a scholarship from FCT.

Conflicts of Interest: The authors declare no conflict of interest.

References

1. Silva, L.C.e.; Fragoso, I.; Teles, J. Injury Profile in Portuguese Children and Adolescents According to Their Level of Sports Participation. *J. Sport Med. Phys. Fit.* **2018**, *58*, 271–279.
2. Silva, L.C.e.; Fragoso, M.I.; Teles, J. Physical Activity–Related Injury Profile in Children and Adolescents According to Their Age, Maturation, and Level of Sports Participation. *Sports Health* **2017**, *9*, 118–125. [CrossRef]
3. Maffulli, N.; Caine, D. The Epidemiology of Children's Team Sports Injuries. *Med. Sport Sci.* **2005**, *49*, 1–8. [PubMed]
4. Van der Sluis, A.; Elferink-Gemser, M.T.; Coelho-e-Silva, M.J.M.; Nijboer, J.A.J.; Brink, M.S.M.; Visscher, C. Sport Injuries Aligned to Peak Height Velocity in Talented Pubertal Soccer Players. *Int. J. Sports Med.* **2014**, *35*, 351–355. [CrossRef] [PubMed]
5. Swenson, D.M.; Henke, N.M.; Collins, C.L.; Fields, S.K.; Comstock, R.D. Epidemiology of United States High School Sports-Related Fractures, 2008–09 to 2010–11. *Am. J. Sports Med.* **2012**, *40*, 2078–2084. [CrossRef] [PubMed]
6. DiFiori, J. Overuse injuries in children and adolescents. *Curr. Sport Med. Rep.* **2010**, *9*, 372–378. [CrossRef] [PubMed]

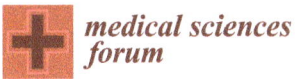

Proceeding Paper

Coffee in the Workplace: A Social Break or a Performance Enhancer? †

Carla F. Rodrigues [1,2,*], Hélder Raposo [1,3], Elsa Pegado [1] and Ana I. Fernandes [4]

1. ISCTE—Instituto Universitário de Lisboa, CIES-ISCTE, 1649-026 Lisboa, Portugal; helder.raposo@estesl.ipl.pt (H.R.); elsa.pegado@iscte-iul.pt (E.P.)
2. Department of Anthropology, Amsterdam Institute for Social Science Research, University of Amsterdam, 1018 WV Amsterdam, The Netherlands
3. ESTeSL-IPL—Escola Superior de Tecnologia da Saúde de Lisboa, Instituto Politécnico de Lisboa, 1990-096 Lisboa, Portugal
4. CiiEM, Interdisciplinary Research Center Egas Moniz, Instituto Universitário Egas Moniz, 2829-511 Almada, Portugal; aifernandes@egasmoniz.edu.pt
* Correspondence: carla.rodrigues@iscte-iul.pt
† Presented at the 5th International Congress of CiiEM—Reducing Inequalities in Health and Society, Online, 16–18 June 2021.

Abstract: Coffee is a socially rooted drink with pharmacological properties. It is embedded in different everyday rituals, including 'coffee breaks' during working hours. This paper analyzes the role of coffee at workplace. Focusing on three professional areas associated with high pressure and responsive demands, we explore the social expression of coffee use at work, and how it is mobilized as a tool for managing sleepiness, fatigue, stress, and concentration problems, amongst other work-related issues.

Keywords: coffee; caffeine; workplace; performance management

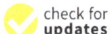

Citation: Rodrigues, C.F.; Raposo, H.; Pegado, E.; Fernandes, A.I. Coffee in the Workplace: A Social Break or a Performance Enhancer? *Med. Sci. Forum* **2021**, *5*, 44. https://doi.org/10.3390/msf2021005044

Academic Editors: Helena Barroso and Cidália Castro

Published: 27 July 2021

Publisher's Note: MDPI stays neutral with regard to jurisdictional claims in published maps and institutional affiliations.

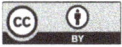

Copyright: © 2021 by the authors. Licensee MDPI, Basel, Switzerland. This article is an open access article distributed under the terms and conditions of the Creative Commons Attribution (CC BY) license (https://creativecommons.org/licenses/by/4.0/).

1. Introduction

As a common beverage in many societies, daily coffee consumption is embedded in different social rituals [1], including the 'coffee breaks' routines at workplace. Besides being a socially rooted drink, coffee's main bioactive compound (caffeine) is claimed to have cognitive enhancing properties associated with fatigue reduction and improvement of mental alertness, concentration, and short-term memory, amongst other performative effects and benefits [2]. Yet, the effect of chronic coffee consumption on the brain is currently starting to be studied [3]. In a context of increasingly competitive economies, where the work rhythms and performance demands are extremely high in many professional environments, what is the role of coffee in managing everyday imperatives at work? Focusing on individuals working in three professional areas—public security, social communication, and healthcare—associated with high pressure and responsive demands, this paper explores the social expression of the use of this stimulant, and how it is mobilized to deal with various issues, including sleepiness, fatigue, stress, and concentration problems.

2. Materials and Methods

This paper draws on an ongoing sociological study on 'performance consumptions' at work, i.e., the use of medicines, food supplements, and other products to improve physical, intellectual, and social performance in the workplace, in Portugal. The analysis presented below is based on qualitative data from seven focus group discussions with a total of 33 participants, and on the interim results of a quantitative survey applied to workers from the three professional areas mentioned above (n = 406). The study was approved by the ethics committee of Egas Moniz and all the participants gave informed written consent to contribute.

3. Results and Discussion

A major critical aspect identified across all professions relates to a time dimension. This regards not only the high number of working hours but also the intensive pace of work, the predominance of irregular working hours (mainly due to rotating shift systems or flexible schedules), multitasking, and the need to quickly adapt to new practices and routines. According to the survey, almost half of the respondents work more than eight hours a day, 40% accumulate different professional activities, and 50% work night shifts. Thus, unsurprisingly, most respondents consider their work rhythms as very, or excessively, intense. Overall, professional demands are high in different domains, particularly concerning intellectual (concentration, mental agility, memorization) and relational (emotional control, communication, conflict management) performance. This has implications on sleep patterns, both in terms of quantity and quality of sleep, which, in turn, also affects work performance—as a vicious cycle.

In these highly demanding professional environments, the pressure for both intellectual and relational performance often leads to the adoption of different strategies to manage stress, increase alertness, improve concentration, and be more productive. In these working contexts, coffee appears as a central resource in managing everyday work performance. According to the survey, 86% of the respondents usually drink coffee on a daily basis. Most coffee users drink up to four cups a day, but, in some cases, intake is much higher. Such high consumption (i.e., five or more coffees daily) is particularly expressive among participants who work for long hours (especially those working 9 to 12 h a day, 49%), who work night shifts (77%), and/or who have other complementary professional activities (47%). Despite the known potential side effects of coffee, where high doses (more than 400mg, cf. EFSA [4]) not only exceed the beneficial ceiling that has been reported as effective for certain performance purposes but may also negatively affect the very concerns caffeine is aimed to address (e.g., increasing anxiety [3]), there is a general reliance on drinking coffee, more than, for instance, on using medicines or food supplements for similar purposes. Among other aspects, the broad acceptance of such a daily consumption practice is linked to its ambivalent social status, as both a substance with pharmacological properties and a common beverage both inside and outside work. While most coffee users' main goal is to stay awake during working hours, more than a third of the survey respondents use it with the aim of having a short break during working time. These coffee breaks are described as moments to decompress, to stretch out the body, to get fresh ideas, and, many times, to socialize with colleagues—which may, as well, have a positive impact on both intellectual and relational performance.

Such multifaceted purposes of coffee use—both social and functional—and its social legitimacy in performance management makes it a privileged tool for managing increasingly fundamental aspects of professional life, which needs further research.

Institutional Review Board Statement: The study was conducted according to the guidelines of the Declaration of Helsinki, and approved by the Ethics Committee of Egas Moniz (protocol code CE 857, approved on the 20 February 2020).

Informed Consent Statement: Informed consent was obtained from all subjects involved in the study.

Data Availability Statement: The data presented are not publicly available, as this was not included in the informed consent obtained from study participants.

Acknowledgments: This study is based on part of a larger research project titled "Medicines and dietary supplements in performance consumptions: social practices, contexts and literacy" (PTDC/SOC-SOC/30734/2017), financed by the Portuguese Foundation for Science and Technology (FCT).

Conflicts of Interest: The authors declare no conflict of interest.

References

1. Giddens, A. *Sociology*, 4th ed.; Polity Press: Cambridge, UK, 2001.
2. Glade, M.J. Caffeine-Not just a stimulant. *Nutrition* **2010**, *26*, 932–938. [CrossRef] [PubMed]

3. Magalhães, R.; Picó-Pérez, M.; Esteves, M.; Vieira, R.; Castanho, T.C.; Amorim, L.; Sousa, M.; Coelho, A.; Fernandes, H.M.; Cabral, J.; et al. Habitual coffee drinkers display a distinct pattern of brain functional connectivity. *Mol. Psychiatry* **2021**. [CrossRef] [PubMed]
4. EFSA. Scientific Opinion on the safety of caffeine. *EFSA J.* **2015**, *13*, 4102. [CrossRef]

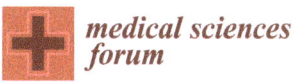

Proceeding Paper

In Vitro Comparative Study of Microhardness and Flexural Strength of Acrylic Resins Used in Removable Dentures [†]

Marta Costa [1,*], Sara Neves [1], Joana Carvalho [1], Sofia Arantes-Oliveira [2] and Sérgio Félix [1,3]

1. Departamento de Reabilitação Oral, Instituto Universitário Egas Moniz, 2829-511 Almada, Portugal; nevessara98@gmail.com (S.N.); joanapscarvalho@gmail.com (J.C.); sfelix1050@gmail.com (S.F.)
2. Faculdade de Medicina Dentária, Universidade de Lisboa, Rua Professora Teresa Ambrósio, Cidade Universitária, 1600-277 Lisboa, Portugal; sofiaaol@fmd.ulisboa.pt
3. Centro de Investigação Interdisciplinar Egas Moniz (CiiEM), Instituto Universitário Egas Moniz, 2829-511 Almada, Portugal
* Correspondence: marta.leonor@hotmail.com
† Presented at the 5th International Congress of CiiEM—Reducing Inequalities in Health and Society, Online, 16–18 June 2021.

Abstract: Polymethylmethacrylate is the material of choice for prosthetic bases. Depending on the type of polymerization, acrylic resins may present some mechanical weaknesses that may lead to the failure of a prosthesis. The microhardness and flexural strength of a dental material determine its applicability. The objective of the present investigation was to evaluate the in vitro Knoop microhardness and flexural strength of a thermopolymerizable (Probase Hot) and an autopolymerizable (Probase Cold) resin, according to ISO 20759-1: 2013.

Keywords: denture; acrylic resins; polymerization; microhardness; flexural strength

1. Introduction

Acrylic resins based on polymethylmethacrylate (PMMA) are obtained by the polymerization of the methylmethacrylate monomer and can be divided into two large groups: "heat-cured" or thermopolymerizable, when polymerization starts with heat, and "cold-cured" or autopolymerizable, when they are chemically activated [1].

Despite some desirable characteristics, PMMA also has some mechanical weaknesses that can lead to fracture, making its ability to resist to fracture a very important parameter that must be be evaluated, specifically, through microhardness and three-point bending tests [2,3].

2. Materials and Methods

Respecting the manufacturer's standards and in accordance with ISO 20759-1: 2013 [4], a total of 10 rectangular specimens of PMMA-based resin were made, i.e., 5 of Probase Hot (PBH) resin and 5 of Probase Cold (PBC) resin, with dimensions of 64 × 10 × 3.3 mm. The specimens were polished with 500 and 100 grain silicon carbide sandpaper and then cooled to room temperature. The specimens were stored in water and incubated at the temperature of 37 ± 1 °C for 48 ± 2 h. The microhardness of each sample was determined using the Knoop test through a Knoop indenter connected to a microhardness machine. In each sample, five indentations were made that the program converted to Knoop microhardness values expressed in kg/mm^2, obtaining the average values. For flexural strength evaluation, the specimens were submitted to the three-point bending test, performed on a universal servo-hydraulic testing machine. Each specimen was tested, applying a distance between the supports of 50 mm and a load to the center of each specimen, using a cross speed of 5 mm/min. Then, the values of the individual measurements (width and thickness) for each specimen were entered into the machine software. Finally, the load was applied, following guidelines from other similar studies until the specimen was fractured, and the fracture load value was recorded in Newton (N). The results obtained were analyzed and compared with a *t*-test, using SPSS software.

3. Results and Discussion

The results obtained through the microhardness test and the three-point bending test (Figure 1) showed significant differences ($p < 0.001$) for the resins under study (Figure 2).

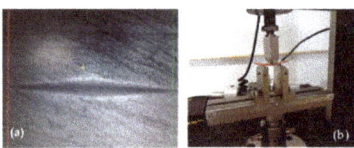

Figure 1. Tests: (**a**) Knoop indentation visualized with an optical microscope; (**b**) three-point bending test.

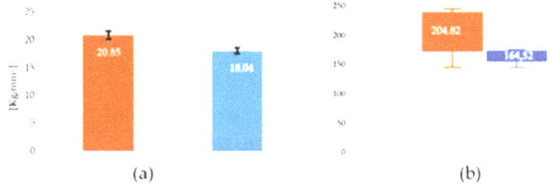

Figure 2. Mechanical characteristics of Probase Hot (orange) and Probase Cold (blue) acrylic resins measured by (**a**) the Knoop microhardness test and (**b**) the three-point bending test.

Thus, within the limitations of this study, the PBH resin presented higher microhardness and flexural strength values than the PBC resin. Scientific evidence demonstrates that autopolymerizable acrylic resins have a lower degree of polymerization. Incomplete polymerization in highly porous structures reduces the physical and mechanical quality of resins [5]. Therefore, this may explain the lower microhardness and flexural strength of PBC.

Institutional Review Board Statement: Not applicable.

Informed Consent Statement: Not applicable.

Data Availability Statement: The data required to reproduce these findings cannot be shared at this time as the data also forms part of an ongoing study.

Conflicts of Interest: The authors declare no conflict of interest.

References

1. Cervino, G.; Cicciù, M.; Herford, A.S.; Germanà, A.; Fiorillo, L. Biological and Chemo-Physical Features of Denture Resin. *Materials* **2020**, *13*, 3350. [CrossRef] [PubMed]
2. Ozkir, S.E.; Yilmaz, B.; Unal, S.M.; Culhaoglu, A.; Kurkcuoglu. Effect of heat polymerization conditions and microwave on the flexural strength of polymethylmethacrylate. *Eur. J. Dent.* **2018**, *12*, 116–119. [CrossRef] [PubMed]
3. Camacho, D.; Svidzinki, T.; Furlaneto, M.; Lopes, M.; Corrêa, G. Acrylic resins for dental use based polymethylmethacrylate. *Braz. J. Surg. Clin. Res.* **2014**, *6*, 63–72. [CrossRef]
4. ISO 20795-1. *Dentistry—Base Polymers—Part 1: Denture Base Polymers*; International Organization for Standardization: Geneva, Switzerland, 2013.
5. Kostic, M.; Petrovic, M.; Krunic, N.; Igic, M.; Janosevic, P. Comparative analysis of water sorption by different acrylic materials. *Acta Med. Median.* **2014**, *53*, 5–9. [CrossRef]

Proceeding Paper

Long-Term Intestinal Failure and Home Parenteral Nutrition: A Single Center Experience †

Mafalda Padinha [1,2,*], Cátia Oliveira [2], Sandra Carlos [2], Ana Paula Santos [2], Marta Brito [2], Carla Adriana Santos [2] and Jorge Fonseca [1,2]

1. PaMNEC—Grupo de Patologia Médica, Nutrição e Exercício Clínico, Centro de Investigação Interdisciplinar Egas Moniz, 2829-511 Almada, Portugal; jorgedafonseca@hotmail.com
2. Hospital Garcia de Orta, 2805-267 Almada, Portugal; sofi.doliveira@gmail.com (C.O.); sandra.carlos@gmail.com (S.C.); apls@netcabo.pt (A.P.S.); marta.brito@hgo.min-saude.pt (M.B.); carla.adriana.santos@hotmail.com (C.A.S.)
* Correspondence: mafaldapadinha98@gmail.com
† Presented at the 5th International Congress of CiiEM—Reducing Inequalities in Health and Society, Online, 16–18 June 2021.

Abstract: Intestinal failure is the reduction in gut function below the minimum necessary for the absorption of macronutrients and/or water electrolytes. The based treatment for type II and III intestinal failure patients is home parenteral nutrition (HPN) and hydration (HPH). This is a case-series study of HPN/HPH patients of the Hospital Garcia de Orta, Portugal, where thirteen patients present different underlying disorders and various IVS needs of nutrition and/or hydration. Most presented type III failure and most of them survived a long period under HPN and/or HNH.

Keywords: intestinal failure; parenteral nutrition; parenteral hydration

1. Introduction

The European Society for Clinical Nutrition and Metabolism (ESPEN) defines intestinal failure as the reduction in gut function below the minimum necessary for the absorption of macronutrients and/or water and electrolytes, such that intravenous supplementation (IVS) is required to maintain health and/or growth [1]. On a pathophysiological perspective, intestinal failure might be divided in three types: type I, short term, with IVS over a period of days/weeks; type II, a long-term subacute condition where IVS is maintained for weeks/months; type III, a chronic condition, in which IVS is required over months/years [2]. Conversely, the clinical classification is based on the IVS requirements of energy and volume; from A to D as the energy IVS, and from 1 to 4 as the volume of the IVS [1]. Although oral nutrient intake is possible in most individuals with intestinal failure, home parenteral nutrition (HPN) and/or hydration (HPH) remain the base of treatment, to prevent malabsorption-associated morbidity. Intestinal failure patients with type II and type III need a multi-disciplinary care, which is given in the Hospital Garcia de Orta. The aim of this study is to evaluate the effectiveness of HPN and HPH in the treatment and prognostic of intestinal failure.

2. Materials and Methods

This study was a case-series study of HPN/HPH patients of the Hospital Garcia de Orta, Almada, Portugal. All clinical files of long-term HPN/HPH patients were selected. The only exclusion criteria was an incomplete file. The present study is a sub-analysis of a large study approved by the ethical committee and the administration of our hospital.

3. Results and Discussion

This study is based on the data of thirteen clinical files, organized and presented in Table 1.

Table 1. Thirteen patients were eligible for this study and classified under the aforementioned criteria.

Patient	Sex	Age	Weight Initial	Weight Final	Underlying Disorders	Pathophysiological Classification	Functional Classification	Clinical Classification	HPH/HPN	Outcome
B.P.	M	71	46.9	54.4	Colon cancer	Short bowel	type III	D2	HPN	Deceased
P.S.	F	84	45	60	intestinal embolism	Short bowel	type III	D2	HPN	Deceased
I.D.	M	65	63	73	Crohn disease	Short bowel + intestinal fistula	type II	D2	HPN	Alive with no IVS
C.J.	M	68	83	87	Colon Cancer	Short bowel	type III	A2	HPH	Deceased
B.S.	M	69	47	76	Familial amyloidotic polyneuropathy	Short bowel	type III	A2	HPH	Alive with IVS
M.G.	F	58	53.8	47.3	Malabsorption from rituximab	Extensive bowel mucosal disease	type III	D2	HPN	Deceased
M.C.	F	63	66.3	72	occlusion surgery	Short bowel + obstruction	type III	A2	HPH	Alive with IVS
M.C.G.	F	92	43.5	52	umbilical hernia	Short bowel	type III	D2	HPN	Deceased
R.S.	F	83	62.9	71	hernioplasty prosthesis fistula	Intestinal fistula	type II	D2	HPN	Alive with no IVS
C.B.	F	62	57	43.3	Intestinal dysmotility	Intestinal dysmotility	type III	D2	HPN	Alive with no IVS
J.L.	M	28	51.7	70.9	Crohn's disease	Short bowel	type III	D2	HPN	Alive with IVS
C.C.	F	47	53	68.1	Gynecological cancer surgery	Short bowel	type III	D2	HPN	Alive with IVS
J.R.	M	43	65	72	F. adenomatous polyposis	Short bowel	type III	A2	HPH	Alive with IVS

Most patients presented type III failure and the majority survived the home parenteral nutrition and/or hydration long period, therefore indicating that these, in fact, are effective forms of treatment for intestinal failure. The deaths observed were most likely due to concomitant morbidities.

Institutional Review Board Statement: Not applicable.

Informed Consent Statement: Not applicable.

Data Availability Statement: Not applicable.

Conflicts of Interest: The authors declare no conflict of interest.

References

1. Pironi, L.; Arends, J.; Baxter, J.; Bozzetti, F.; Peláez, R.B.; Cuerda, C.; Forbes, A.; Gabe, S.; Gillanders, L.; Holst, M.; et al. ESPEN endorsed recommendations. Definition and classification of intestinal failure in adults. *Clin. Nutr.* **2015**, *34*, 171–180. [CrossRef] [PubMed]
2. Pironi, L.; Arends, J.; Bozzetti, F.; Cuerda, C.; Gillanders, L.; Jeppesen, P.B.; Joly, F.; Kelly, D.; Lal, S.; Staun, M.; et al. ESPEN guidelines on chronic intestinal failure in adults. *Clin. Nutr.* **2016**, *35*, 247–307. [CrossRef] [PubMed]

MDPI
St. Alban-Anlage 66
4052 Basel
Switzerland
Tel. +41 61 683 77 34
Fax +41 61 302 89 18
www.mdpi.com

Medical Sciences Editorial Office
E-mail: medsci@mdpi.com
www.mdpi.com/journal/medsci

www.ingramcontent.com/pod-product-compliance
Lightning Source LLC
LaVergne TN
LVHW070559100526
838202LV00012B/507